**W9-CHF-423**

# Your *Clinics* subscription just got better!

## You can now access the FULL TEXT of this publication online at no additional cost! Activate your online subscription today and receive...

- Full text of all issues from 2002 to the present
- Photographs, tables, illustrations, and references
- Comprehensive search capabilities
- Links to MEDLINE and Elsevier journals

**Activate Your Online Access Today!**

Plus, you can also sign up for E-alerts of upcoming issues or articles that interest you, and take advantage of exclusive access to bonus features!

## To activate your individual online subscription:

1. Visit our website at **www.TheClinics.com**.

2. Click on "Register" at the top of the page, and follow the instructions.

3. To activate your account, you will need your subscriber account number, which you can find on your mailing label (note: the number of digits in your subscriber account number varies from six to ten digits). See the sample below where the subscriber account number has been circled.

**This is your subscriber account number**

```
************************************3-DIGIT 001
FEB00   J0167   C7   123456-89   10/00   Q: 1

J.H. DOE, MD
531 MAIN ST
CENTER CITY, NY  10001-001
```

4. That's it! Your online access to the most trusted source for clinical reviews is now available.

# theclinics.com

ELSEVIER

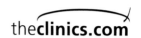

# CARDIOLOGY CLINICS

Therapeutic Strategies in Diabetes
and Cardiovascular Disease

GUEST EDITOR
Prakash C. Deedwania, MD, FACC, FACP, FCCP, FAHA

CONSULTING EDITOR
Michael H. Crawford, MD

May 2005 • Volume 23 • Number 2

**SAUNDERS**

An Imprint of Elsevier, Inc.
PHILADELPHIA   LONDON   TORONTO   MONTREAL   SYDNEY   TOKYO

**W.B. SAUNDERS COMPANY**

*A Division of Elsevier Inc.*

The Curtis Center • Independence Square West • Philadelphia, Pennsylvania 19106

http://www.theclinics.com

**CARDIOLOGY CLINICS**
May 2005
Editor: Karen Sorensen

Volume 23, Number 2
ISSN 0733-8651
ISBN 1-4160-2699-1

Reprints. For copies of 100 or more, of articles in this publication, please contact the Commercial Reprints Department, Elsevier Inc., 360 Park Avenue South, New York, New York 10010-1710. Tel. (212) 633-3813 Fax: (212) 462-1935 email: reprints@elsevier.com

The ideas and opinions expressed in *Cardiology Clinics* do not necessarily reflect those of the Publisher. The Publisher does not assume any responsibility for any injury and/or damage to persons or property arising out of or related to any use of the material contained in this periodical. The reader is advised to check the appropriate medical literature and the product information currently provided by the manufacturer of each drug to be administered to verify the dosage, the method and duration of administration, or contraindications. It is the responsibility of the treating physician or other health care professional, relying on independent experience and knowledge of the patient, to determine drug dosages and the best treatment for the patient. Mention of any product in this issue should not be construed as endorsement by the contributors, editors, or the Publisher of the product or manufacturers' claims.

*Cardiology Clinics* (ISSN 0733-8651) is published quarterly by W.B. Saunders Company; Corporate and editorial Offices: The Curtis Center, Independence Square West, Philadelphia, PA 19106-3399. Accounting and circulation offices: 6277 Sea Harbor Drive, Orlando, FL 32887-4800. Periodicals postage paid at Orlando, FL 32862, and additional mailing offices. Subscription prices are $170.00 per year for US individuals, $266.00 per year for US institutions, $85.00 per year for US students and residents, $210.00 per year for Canadian individuals, $323.00 per year for Canadian institutions, $230.00 per year for international individuals, $323.00 per year for international institutions and $115.00 per year for Canadian and foreign students/residents. To receive student/resident rate, orders must be accompanied by name of affiliated institution, data of term, and the *signature* of program/residency coordinator on institution letterhead. Orders will be billed at individual rate until proof of status is received. Foreign air speed delivery is included in all *Clinics* subscription prices. All prices are subject to change without notice. POSTMASTER: Send address changes to *Cardiology Clinics*, W.B. Saunders Company, Periodicals Fulfillment, Orlando, FL 32887-4800. **Customer Service: 1-800-654-2452 (US). From outside of the US, call 1-407-345-1000.**

*Cardiology Clinics* is also published in Spanish by McGraw-Hill Interamericana Editores S. A., P.O. Box 5-237, 06500, Mexico D. F., Mexico; in Portuguese by Reichmann and Alfonso Editores Rio de Janeiro, Brazil; and in Greek by Dimitrios P. Lagos, 8 Pondon Street, GR115-28 Ilissia, Greece.

*Cardiology Clinics* is covered in *Index Medicus, Excerpta Medica, The Cumulative Index to Nursing and Allied Health Literature* (INAHL).

# CONSULTING EDITOR

**MICHAEL H. CRAWFORD, MD,** Professor, Department of Medicine, University of California Medical School; and Chief of Clinical Cardiology, Division of Cardiology, University of California, San Francisco, San Francisco, California

# GUEST EDITOR

**PRAKASH C. DEEDWANIA, MD, FACC, FACP, FCCP, FAHA,** Professor, Department of Medicine, University of California, San Francisco School of Medicine, San Francisco; Chief, Cardiology Section, Veterans Administration Central California Health Care System/University of California Program, Fresno; Director, Cardiovascular Research, UCSF Program, Fresno; and Clinical Professor of Medicine, Stanford University, Palo Alto, California

# CONTRIBUTORS

**JOHN B. BUSE, MD, PhD,** Associate Professor, Medicine, Division of Endocrinology; Chief, Division of General Medicine and Clinical Epidemiology; and Director, Diabetes Care Center, University of North Carolina School of Medicine, Chapel Hill, North Carolina

**VIVIAN A. FONSECA, MD,** Professor, Departments of Medicine and Pharmacology, Tullis-Tulane Alumni Chair in Diabetes; Director, Tulane Diabetes Program, Tulane University Medical Center, New Orleans; and Department of Medicine, Veterans Affairs Medical Center, New Orleans, Louisiana

**OM P. GANDA, MD,** Director of the Lipid Clinic, Joslin Diabetes Center; Associate Clinical Professor, Department of Medicine, Harvard Medical School; and Attending Physician, Department of Endocrinology and Metabolism, Beth-Israel Deaconess Medical Center, Boston, Massachusetts

**ALI A. JAWA, MD,** Assistant Professor, Department of Medicine, Tulane University Medical Center, New Orleans; and Department of Medicine, Veterans Affairs Medical Center, New Orleans, Louisiana

**DEBABRATA MUKHERJEE, MD, MS, FACC,** Tyler Gill Professor, Interventional Cardiology; Director, Peripheral Intervention Program; and Associate Director, Cardiac Catheterization Laboratories, Gill Heart Institute, Division of Cardiovascular Medicine, University of Kentucky, Lexington, Kentucky

**JULIO ROSENSTOCK, MD,** Dallas Diabetes and Endocrine Center; and Clinical Professor, Medicine, University of Texas Southwestern Medical School, Dallas, Texas

**SUNDARARAJAN SRIKANTH, MD,** Assistant Clinical Professor, Department of Medicine, Veterans Administration Central California Health Care System/University Medical Center, University of California, San Francisco Program at Fresno, Fresno, California

**KRIS VIJAYARAGHAVAN, MD,** Director of Research and Heart Failure Program, Scottsdale Cardiovascular Research Institute, Scottsdale; Director, Congestive Heart Failure Clinic, Arizona Heart Hospital; and Clinical Professor of Medicine, Midwestern Osteopathic School of Medicine, Glendale, Arizona

**STUART W. ZARICH, MD, FACC,** Chairman, Division of Cardiovascular Medicine, Bridgeport Hospital; and Assistant Clinical Professor of Medicine, Yale University School of Medicine, Bridgeport, Connecticut

# CONTENTS

disease. Thiazide diuretics and calcium-channel blockers are the second-line drugs. Angiotensin II-receptor blockers may prove to be as effective as ACE inhibitors in diabetics who have hypertension. α-Adrenergic antagonists should be avoided. Most hypertensive patients require more than one agent to control their blood pressure. There is no evidence to support one combination regimen over others; however, the combination of ACE-I with a thiazide diuretic or a β-blocker may be the most cost effective regimen.

# FORTHCOMING ISSUES

# RECENT ISSUES

---

## VISIT OUR WEB SITE

The Clinics are now available online!
**Access your subscription at www.theclinics.com**

---

ELSEVIER
SAUNDERS

Cardiol Clin 23 (2005) ix

CARDIOLOGY
CLINICS

Foreword

# Therapeutic Strategies in Diabetes and Cardiovascular Disease

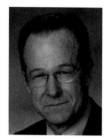

Michael H. Crawford, MD
*Consulting Editor*

Diabetes is now considered the equivalent of having 2 or 3 major risk factors for coronary atherosclerosis. Also, the presence of diabetes increases the risk of any procedure and is associated with a poorer prognosis compared with individuals without diabetes. Also, diabetes dictates certain clinical approaches to disease. Thus today's clinician needs a full understanding of this disease and its effect on management decisions.

I was delighted that Dr. Prakash Deedwania, who has had a long and productive interest in diabetes and cardiovascular disease, was willing to organize and contribute to articles on this topic. This broad topic has been divided between two issues of the *Cardiology Clinics*. The first issue (November 2004) dealt with pathophysiology, clinical epidemiology, and the relationship between diabetes and other diseases such as heart failure and hypertension. The second issue deals with management strategies for preventing and treating the cardiovascular complications of diabetes. I am indebted to Dr. Deedwania and the group of experts he has assembled for these two important issues. Editing one issue is a big job, let alone two. However, Dr. Deedwania has had a long-standing academic and clinical interest in diabetes and metabolic syndrome in cardiovascular disease. His dedication to improving care for these individuals is evident in these two issues of the *Cardiology Clinics*.

Michael H. Crawford, MD
*Division of Cardiology*
*University of California*
*505 Parnassus Ave., Box 0124*
*San Francisco, CA 94143-0124, USA*

*E-mail address:* crawfordm@medicine.ucsf.edu

Preface

# Therapeutic Strategies in Diabetes and Cardiovascular Disease

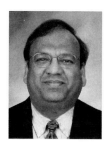

Prakash C. Deedwania, MD, FACC, FACP, FCCP, FAHA
*Guest Editor*

Cardiovascular (CV) complications are the leading cause of death and disability in patients with type II diabetes mellitus. As described in the November 2004 issue of the *Cariology Clinics*, it is important to recognize that vascular abnormalities and dysfunction begin in the prediabetic phase, which often precedes development of clinical signs and symptoms of diabetes by an average of 5 to 6 years.

Although due emphasis has been placed on tight control of blood glucose in diabetic patients during the past two decades, the management of other frequently associated coronary risk factors has not received as much attention. A large number of randomized clinical trials have now shown that aggressive management of most associated risk factors—in particular hypertension and hyperlipidemia in diabetic patients—is associated with significant reduction of the risk of future CV events. As a matter of fact, beginning with the findings from the United Kingdom Prospective Diabetes studies, many of the trials have demonstrated that tight control of blood pressure is more beneficial in reducing the rate of CV complications in diabetic patients. Similar results are beginning to emerge from the trials with statins in patients with diabetes. Although more work is needed, there is emerging evidence that for maximum CV protection comprehensive risk reduction approach is necessary and feasible. It is also important to

realize that because of the overall increased absolute risk of CV events, diabetic patients tend to benefit more with most of the effective risk factor interventions. Based on the results of these studies, various guideline committees have set aggressive goals for therapy in diabetic patients. However, despite the available evidence and guideline recommendations, most diabetic patients are not at goal blood pressure, target lipid levels, or good long-term glycemic control. Serious medical attention and concerted clinical efforts are needed to achieve adequate control of all risk factors in diabetic patients to provide maximum CV protection. It is also important to realize that such interventions are not only good for these patients, they are cost-effective as well.

It was with the above points in mind and the obvious need to examine the benefits of various treatment options in diabetic patients that this issue of the *Cardiology Clinics* was conceived. Its primary goal is to present state-of-the-art articles that examine and summarize the most relevant literature dealing with treatment of various components that are associated with increased risk of CV complications in diabetes. The authors represent an outstanding group of internationally recognized authorities in their field.

The first article examines the role of intensive glycemic control during the acute phase of acute myocardial infarction in diabetic patients. This is

0733-8651/05/$ - see front matter © 2005 Elsevier Inc. All rights reserved.
doi:10.1016/j.ccl.2004.12.001

followed by an article describing and comparing the role of traditional oral hypoglycemic drugs such as insulin secretagogues and the newer insulin-sensitizing agents in preventing CV complications of diabetes. The next article deals with the common problem of the deadly duet of diabetes and hypertension and describes the totality of evidence demonstrating the benefits of aggressive blood pressure reduction in reducing the rate of coronary events, congestive heart failure, strokes, and renal complications in patients with diabetes.

It is now well recognized that many diabetic patients have atherogenic dyslipidemia. A number of recent clinical trials have also documented the benefits of lipid-lowering therapies in diabetic patients. The article by Ganda provides a critical appraisal regarding various issues dealing with lipid abnormalities and management considerations in diabetes. The best approach for prevention of CV complications in diabetes would be prevention of diabetes itself, and it is with this point in mind that the next article in the issue describes the preventive strategies with special emphasis on the emerging evidence suggesting potential benefits of renal-angiotensin system blockade in the prevention of diabetes and the related CV complications.

Ever since the results of the bypass angioplasty revascularization investigation trial became available there has been considerable controversy regarding the most appropriate revascularization strategy in diabetic patients. The article by Mukherjee provides a comprehensive review regarding the role of percutaneous coronary intervention versus coronary artery bypass graft surgery in diabetes. Finally, as stated earlier, there is emerging evidence that to achieve the maximum benefits of therapeutic strategy, a comprehensive risk reduction approach that incorporates aggressive risk factor modification is necessary. The article by Srikant and Deedwania provides a critical appraisal and clinically meaningful ideas to incorporate an integrated approach for comprehensive CV risk reduction in diabetes. The last article in the issue provides the rationale and summary of various clinical trials examining a variety of therapeutic approaches for the prevention of CV complications in diabetes.

It is my hope that the compendium of articles in this issue spanning from established therapies to emerging treatments and therapeutic approaches in the future will help clinicians achieve the goal of providing maximum CV protection to patients with diabetes.

I would like to thank Michael Crawford, MD, the Consulting Editor of the *Cardiology Clinics*, for inviting me to compile this second issue dealing with diabetes and CV disease. I would especially like to express my gratitude to all of the contributors and collaborators for providing their input and articles in a timely manner. Finally, I would like to thank my family and friends, who are always so supportive of my academic endeavors.

Prakash C. Deedwania, MD,
FACC, FACP, FCCP, FAHA
*Veterans Administration*
*Central California*
*Health Care System*
*University of California–San Francisco at Fresno*
*2615 E. Clinton Avenue*
*Fresno, CA 93703, USA*

*E-mail address:* deed@ucsfresno.edu

CARDIOLOGY
CLINICS

Cardiol Clin 23 (2005) 109–117

# The Role of Intensive Glycemic Control in the Management of Patients who have Acute Myocardial Infarction

Stuart W. Zarich, MD, FACC

*Division of Cardiovascular Medicine, Department of Medicine, Bridgeport Hospital,*
*267 Grant Street, Bridgeport, CT 06610, USA*
*Yale University School of Medicine, 333 Cedar Street, New Haven, CT 06510, USA*

Individuals who have diabetes mellitus (DM) have a twofold to fourfold increased risk of cardiovascular disease and nearly twice the early mortality from acute myocardial infarction (AMI) compared with nondiabetic subjects [1–5]. Furthermore, the mortality difference between diabetics and nondiabetics continues to increase throughout the first year [4]. For more than 70 years it has been recognized that glucosuria is present frequently in nondiabetic patients who have AMI [6]. Acute hyperglycemia is documented in up to half of all patients who have AMI, whereas previously diagnosed DM is present in only 20% to 25% of these patients [7,8].

Elevated plasma glucose and glycated hemoglobin levels at admission are recognized as independent prognosticators of in-hospital and long-term cardiovascular events in diabetics and nondiabetics who have AMI [8–12]. Acute hyperglycemia is associated with an approximate fourfold risk of death with AMI in nondiabetics compared with a nearly twofold increased risk of death in diabetic individuals [10].

It is not clear whether "stress hyperglycemia" predisposes one to a worse prognosis or is simply a marker for more extensive myocardial damage. Acute hyperglycemia in AMI probably is not related simply to stress-mediated release of counterregulatory hormones (catecholamines, glucagon, and cortisol) because glucose levels that are measured upon hospital admission do not correlate necessarily with the extent of myocardial damage as measured by myocardial enzyme release [9,13]. A large, randomized, controlled trial in diabetics who had AMI showed that reduced short- and long-term mortality in low- and high-risk subjects was associated with lowering plasma glucose with insulin [14–16]. This suggests that hyperglycemia is not just a passive by-product of the stress response in the most critically ill patients. Low-risk diabetic individuals and those who had previous insulin use benefited the most from aggressive management of hyperglycemia.

An alternative explanation for the relationship between glucose levels that are measured upon hospital admission and prognosis is the link between insulin resistance, the metabolic syndrome, and cardiovascular (CV) disease. Metabolic syndrome is characterized by insulin resistance and the association with traditional (the "deadly quartet" of obesity, hypertension, glucose intolerance, atherogenic dyslipidemia) and novel (endothelial dysfunction, proinflammatory state, hypercoagulability) risk factors for the development of CV disease and DM [17,18]. The metabolic syndrome is present in approximately 30% of middle-aged men [17] and is associated with a threefold to fourfold increase in CV mortality as compared with controls, even when patients who had known CV disease and DM were excluded from analysis [18]. Patients who have insulin resistance and frank DM also may have a host of associated conditions (Box 1) that may contribute to a poor CV prognosis.

*E-mail address:* pszari@bpthosp.org

---

**Box 1. Associated conditions which may help to explain the poor outcome in DM and Insulin resistance**

*Maladaptive left ventricular remodeling of the noninfarct zone*
Influenced by:
    Increased prevalence of silent myocardial infarction
    Automatic neuropathy
    Increased collagen deposition in the myocardium
    Increased endothelial dysfunction that leads to myocardial ischemia

*Diabetic cardiomyopathy*

*Increased severity and extent of coronary artery disease*

*Associated conditions*
Older age and associated comorbidity
Endothelial dysfunction
Autonomic dysfunction (sympathovagal imbalance)
Abnormalities of coagulation, fibrinolysis, platelet function
Other established vascular disease

*Associated features*
Hypertension
Dyslipidemia (increased very low density lipoprotein, triglycerides, and small dense low
    density lipoprotein, low high density lipoprotein)
Obesity
Insulin resistance
Renal disease: microalbuminuria, proteinuria, and nephropathy
Reduced development of coronary collateral vessels

---

Recent data shown that the prevalence of DM or impaired glucose tolerance (IGT) may be as high as 70% in patients who have AMI [19]. In 181 consecutive nondiabetics who had AMI, more than two thirds of patients were diagnosed with DM or IGT by oral glucose tolerance testing. Previously undiagnosed DM accounted for one half of all patients who had AMI and an abnormal glucose metabolism. Only one third of subjects met criteria for DM based on fasting blood glucose criteria. Although a random blood glucose at the time of admission for AMI may not be reliable in making the diagnosis of DM, concern that the diagnosis of IGT or DM is erroneous in the acute setting because of "stress hyperglycemia" may be unwarranted; the results of glucose tolerance testing that was performed at the time of AMI were similar to those performed 3 months later. Two recent studies in patients who presented for coronary angiography similarly showed that previously undiagnosed DM or IGT was present in up to two thirds of patients who had angiographically-proven coronary artery disease [20–21].

Acute hyperglycemia is associated with a myriad of adverse metabolic and CV effects that may contribute to a poor outcome in AMI (Box 2). Exaggerated metabolic responses to ischemia may play a crucial role in myocardial oxygen use in AMI. Hyperglycemia is a reflection of relative insulinopenia, which is associated with increased lipolysis and free fatty acid (FFA) generation, diminished myocardial glucose uptake, and a decrease in glycolytic substrate for myocardial energy needs in AMI [22–24]. Although glucose metabolism is a major myocardial energy source, oxidation of FFAs is the primary source of energy in the resting aerobic state. During myocardial ischemia, FFA oxidation rates decrease but remain an important source of energy. During reperfusion, fatty acid oxidation again dominates as a source of energy.

Myocardial ischemia results in an increased rate of glycogen breakdown and glucose uptake by way of translocation of glucose transport receptors (GLUT-4) to the sarcolemma [25,26]. This adaptive mechanism is important because

---

**Box 2. Acute effects of hyperglycemia in acute myocardial infarction**

Endothelial dysfunction
Platelet hyperreactivity
Increased cytokine activation
Increased lipolysis and FFA levels
Reduced glycolysis and glucose oxidation
Osmotic diuresis (potentially reduced cardiac output)
Increased oxidative stress (? increased myocardial apoptosis)
Impaired microcirculatory function (no reflow phenomenon)
Impaired ischemic preconditioning
Impaired insulin secretion and insulin-stimulated glucose uptake

---

glucose oxidation requires less oxygen than FFA oxidation to maintain ATP production. Thus, myocardial energy use is more efficient during the increased dependence on glucose oxidation with ischemia (approximately 11% more ATP is generated from glucose oxidation as compared with FFA oxidation). In the setting of relative insulinopenia (insulin resistance or frank DM) that is exacerbated by the stress of AMI, the ischemic myocardium is forced to use FFAs more than glucose for an energy source because myocardial glucose uptake is impaired acutely. Thus, despite acute hyperglycemia, a metabolic crisis may ensue as the hypoxic myocardium becomes less energy efficient in the setting of frank DM or insulin resistance.

Insulin augments the translocation of GLUT-1 and GLUT-4 receptors to the sarcolemma and can diminish FFA release from myocytes and adipocytes [27]. Thus, the extent to which the myocardium expresses an intact response to insulin, therapeutic augmentation of oxidative glucose metabolism by way of exogenous insulin, or improved insulin sensitivity may play a useful role for improving outcomes in patients who have hyperglycemia and relative insulinopenia as the result of an insulin-resistant state. The concept of a metabolic cocktail to promote glucose oxidation and reduce FFA levels to protect the ischemic myocardium dates back to Sodi-Pallares et al [28]. Early studies yielded promising results; a subsequent meta-analysis of 1932 patients who had AMI suggested that therapy with glucose-insulin-potassium (GIK) reduced mortality by 28% [29]. Mortality was reduced by 48% in a subgroup of patients who received high-dose GIK to suppress FFA levels maximally. A prominent Latin American Study [30] further suggested that GIK in the setting of acute reperfusion (predominantly thrombolysis) for patients who had AMI reduced in-hospital mortality by 66%. There was a remarkable reduction in absolute mortality of 10% (15.2% to 5.2%) in GIK-treated reperfused patients versus controls.

Despite nearly a half century of study and its low cost and minimal side-effect profile, acceptance of the GIK metabolic cocktail in AMI has not been forthcoming. The lack of enthusiasm over the use of GIK in AMI seems to stem from the lack of large randomized trials, controversy over low- versus high-dose therapy, and a cumbersome mode of delivery that requires a large volume load. Collectively, clinical studies suggest that the dose of insulin must be optimized to confer benefit; little effect is seen with low-dose GIK protocols [30–31]. In addition, GIK studies have contained only a small number of high-risk patients who had congestive heart failure or cardiogenic shock.

Recently, Van der Horst et al [32] reported the results of the largest study to date of GIK in combination with acute reperfusion with primary angioplasty. Overall, in this 940-patient Dutch study, there was no difference in mortality between those who received GIK and those who received placebo (4.8% versus 5.8%; $P = 0.5$). In 856 patients who did not have heart failure, mortality was reduced 72% with GIK as compared with placebo (1.2% versus 4.2%; $P < 0.005$). There was a nonsignificant trend toward benefit in the diabetic subgroup. The prevalence of the highest quartile of infarct size also was reduced among subjects who received GIK (22% versus 29%; $P < 0.005$), with a trend toward a lower prevalence of ejection fractions less than 30% (13% versus 17%; $P = 0.2$) in subjects who received GIK compared with subjects who did not.

GIK was not beneficial, however, in patients who had congestive heart failure in the Dutch study, as compared with a trend toward benefit in the Latin American trial. The sample size of patients who had heart failure was small in both studies and the infusion rate was twice as fast in the Dutch study; this resulted in more than 2 L of fluid being delivered in the first 8 hours. Additionally, successful reperfusion was accomplished in only a modest number of patients who had heart failure in both studies. Outcomes were remarkably similar in GIK-treated patients who did not have heart failure in the aforementioned studies, despite a wide range in the duration of symptoms before GIK therapy (2.5 to 11 hours). To help to address the issues that surround GIK therapy, a large, randomized trial of GIK therapy in AMI is currently in progress (GIK II: http://www.ecla.org.ar).

In the Diabetes Mellitus Insulin Glucose Infusion in Acute Myocardial Infarction (DIGAMI) trial [14–16], acute treatment for at least 24 hours with intravenous GIK until blood sugar was controlled, coupled with aggressive subacute treatment with subcutaneous insulin, resulted in a 29% relative reduction in 1-year mortality in a cohort of patients that predominantly had type 2 DM. As compared with 43% of control patients, 87% of GIK-treated patients were discharged on insulin. Patients who had previous insulin use and a low CV risk profile had the most promising results (58% reduction in in-hospital mortality and 52% reduction in 1-year mortality). Hypoglycemia occurred in 15% of patients who received insulin infusion; however, only 10% of patients required discontinuation of their insulin infusion.

Recently, the results of the DIGAMI-2 trial further highlighted the importance of glucose lowering in AMI. However, this pivotal trial, which was released at the 2004 European Association for the Study of Diabetes, failed to show an improvement in total mortality in diabetic patients with AMI undergoing intensive insulin therapy. The trial was initially designed to include 3000 subjects but was stopped at 1253 subjects due to poor enrollment. DIGAMI-2 compared acute insulin–glucose infusion followed by an insulin-based long-term glucose control with insulin–glucose infusion followed by standard glucose control or routine metabolic management in the third group according to physician discretion.

The results of the DIGAMI-2 trial were confounded by several factors. The actual mortality was significantly lower than the estimated mortality for the group at 2 years, and the mean hemoglobin A1c at the time of enrollment in all three groups was relatively low at 7.3%. The glucose goal was not reached in the intensive therapy group; 41% of patients in the control group with routine care received extra insulin in the hospital, and 14% received insulin infusions. Multidose insulin for glucose lowering was given to only 42% of patients chronically in the intensively managed group (compared with 13%–15% in the two remaining groups). Glucose control over the duration of the study was similar in the three groups (mean hemoglobin A1c: 6.8%). The mortality ranged between 19.3% and 23.4% between the three groups, which was not statistically significant.

There was appropriate use of cardioprotective drugs during AMI in the DIGAMI-2 trial. At hospital discharge, beta-blockers were given to over 80% of the patients, aspirin was given to nearly 90% of the patients, and angiotensin-converting enzyme (ACE) inhibitors and statin therapy were given to approximately 65% of the patients. The overall 2-year mortality of approximately 20%, although significantly lower than the 30% noted in the DIGAMI-1 trial, is evidence that there is still much work to do. Overall these results suggest that the mode of glucose therapy may not matter as much as aggressive glucose control. Because all three groups reached a similar mean A1c of below 7%, the hypothesis of the trial was not fully tested. Additionally, there was significant crossover with the use of both acute intravenous insulin therapy and chronic insulin therapy in the three groups, complicating the analysis of insulin-based therapy compared with the routine use of oral hypoglycemic agents after myocardial infarction.

Acutely GIK therapy decreases lipolysis and improves glucose oxidation; aggressive metabolic therapy also is associated with a myriad of effects in ischemic/reperfused myocardium and in non-infarcted myocardium that is exposed to increased afterload stress (Box 3). FFA levels rapidly increase in AMI as a result of the lipolysis that is secondary to catecholamine excess (and the presence of heparin). FFAs are directly toxic to the myocardium, promote arrhythmogenesis, and, are inefficient as a metabolic substrate. GIK shifts oxidative metabolism from FFA to glucose, lowers circulating FFA levels, and seems to protect myocytes from increasing intracellular calcium levels that are associated with ischemia [33].

> **Box 3. Acute benefits of insulin and glucose therapy in acute myocardial infarction**
>
> Improve glucose oxidation
> Reduce circulating FFA levels
> Vasodilation
> Decrease thromboxane AII levels
> Increase prostacyclin release
> Diminish plasminogen activator
>     inhibitor-1 levels
> "Polarizing effect"—decrease
>     arrhythmogenesis
> Improve endothelial function
> Improve platelet function
> Improve ischemic/nonischemic left
>     ventricular dysfunction
> Replete glycogen pool—protect
>     against reperfusion injury
> ?Protect against increased
>     intracellular calcium levels
> ?Decrease myocardial apoptosis
>     post reperfusion

Adjacent nonischemic myocardium is exposed to an acute pressure load during AMI that resulted, experimentally, in diminished levels of high energy substrate and accelerated ventricular failure [34]. Augmenting glucose oxidation maintained ventricular function in the above murine model of acute pressure during AMI overload. Thus, acutely loaded nonischemic myocardium may benefit markedly from increased glucose uptake and oxidation in the setting of GIK.

Experimental data also support a direct cardioprotective effect of insulin [35–36]. Experimental GIK infusion was equally effective in reducing infarct size when given throughout the entire ischemia/reperfusion cycle or only during reperfusion [37]. Subsequently, insulin attenuated myocardial apoptosis that was associated with reperfusion [38]. Additionally, some of the benefit that was seen in recent trials of insulin therapy in AMI in diabetic subjects may have been due to the withdrawal of sulfonylurea therapy. Although controversial, sulfonylureas block ATP-sensitive potassium channels and may impair ischemic preconditioning and coronary vasodilation and increase mortality in AMI [39–40].

Analogous to the setting of AMI, hyperglycemia in critically-ill subjects is associated with increased complications [41]. Aggressive insulin therapy and control of hyperglycemia also improves outcomes in critically-ill patients in whom withdrawal of sulfonylureas was not a significant factor [42]. Continuous infusion of intravenous insulin to maintain a blood glucose level that was at or less than 110 mg/dL reduced death, septicemia, and renal failure in a predominantly nondiabetic Belgian population of surgical patients who were mechanically-ventilated and critically ill. Aggressive glucose control also reduced complications in diabetic patients who were undergoing cardiac bypass surgery [43–44] and reduced target vessel revascularization in diabetics who were undergoing percutaneous revascularization [45]. Glycemic control also is associated with a decreased risk for congestive heart failure in DM [46].

In support of the "glucometabolic" hypothesis, recent clinical studies demonstrated anti-ischemic effects with newer metabolic agents that improve myocardial energy substrate use [47]. The use of partial fatty acid oxidation inhibitors is the alternative strategy of promoting glucose oxidation that seems to be the most promising in clinical studies. The 3-ketoacyl-coenzyme thiolase inhibitors, trimetazidine and ranolazine, reduced myocardial ischemia in animal and clinical models [48–49]. These compounds work by switching myocardial metabolism from FFAs to glucose oxidation and diminish the decrease of intracellular ATP that occurs during periods of ischemia.

In contrast to the role of insulin therapy, the role of oral hypoglycemic agents in AMI has not been well-studied. Thiazolidinediones significantly reduced infarct size and contractile dysfunction and were beneficial in preventing left ventricular remodeling in experimental models of ischemia/reperfusion [50–52]. Clinical studies in acute ischemia in humans are lacking, however. Chronically, thiazolidenediones improve insulin resistance and have a host of nonhypoglycemic effects that result in improved endothelial and fibrinolytic function and diminished levels of proinflammatory cytokines, high sensitivity-C reactive protein and soluble CD-40 [53–55]. Thiazolidinediones also have direct effects on vascular smooth muscle, may have potent antirestenotic effects [56–57], and were associated with regression of atherosclerosis [58]. Metformin therapy also is associated with a host of salutary effects on CV risk factors [59–60] and may reduce CV events in obese patients who have type 2 DM [61]. The second Bypass Angioplasty Revascularization Investigation will attempt to answer the question whether treatment of DM with insulin-sensitizing agents is preferred over treatment with insulin-providing agents in diabetics who have vascular disease.

Finally, it is important to re-emphasize that, compared with a general population, therapy with primary angioplasty, thrombolysis, β-blockers, aspirin, ACE inhibitors, glycoprotein IIb/IIIa inhibitors, and statins are at least as effective in patients who have DM. Despite this, there is significant underuse of these proven therapies in diabetic patients [62]. Sympathetic blockade inhibits lipolysis and the generation of circulating FFA, which compromises glycolysis in ischemic and nonischemic myocardium. Therefore, it is not surprising that β-blockers are particularly beneficial in diabetic patients. Recently, more complete sympathetic blockage with carvedilol was superior to β-blocker therapy with metoprolol in reducing mortality in patients who had congestive heart failure [63]. Unlike other commercially-available β-blockers, carvedilol therapy improved insulin resistance and may be more effective in reversing left ventricular remodeling by improving myocardial energetics. Although DM is associated with an increase in adverse events in the setting of either percutaneous or surgical revascularization [64], it is clear that diabetics will require coronary intervention; the optimal strategy awaits the results of future studies.

## Summary

Hyperglycemia is associated with excess mortality in AMI and should be treated aggressively in the intensive care setting. The exact goal of therapy is unclear because different blood glucose targets were used in earlier studies (eg, 215 mg/dL in DIGAMI versus 110 mg/dL in the Belgian study of critically-ill patients). In the setting of AMI, it is prudent to avoid excessive hypoglycemia and, thus, more modest goals for blood glucose may be considered until more definitive data are present. Aggressive therapy with continuous infusion of insulin seems to improve a host of metabolic and physiologic effects that are associated with acute hyperglycemia and improves mortality in the acute setting. Aggressive glycemic control should be coupled with appropriate use of reperfusion therapies, glycoprotein IIb/IIIa inhibitors, aspirin, β-blockers, ACE inhibitors, and antithrombotic agents.

The role of intensive chronic glucose control in reducing CV events is less clear but earlier studies
were not well-powered; did not achieve aggressive, durable glycemic control; and did not use insulin-sensitizing agents routinely [65]. Given the results of the DIGAMI trial, the goal of therapy postdischarge should include strict glycemic control while future studies help to delineate the role of insulin-sensitizing agents versus insulin-providing agents in reducing recurrent macrovascular events. Careful attention also should be paid to aggressive lifestyle modifications and treatment of hypertension, hyperlipidemia, and left ventricular dysfunction, as well as appropriate use of antiplatelet and antithrombotic agents.

## References

[1] Stamler J, Vaccaro O, Neaton JD, Wentworth D. For the Multiple Risk Factor Intervention Trail Research Group. Diabetes, other risk factors and 12-year cardiovascular mortality for men screened in the Multiple Risk Factor Invention Trial. Diabetes Care 1993;16:434–44.

[2] Kannel W. Lipids, diabetes, and coronary heart disease: insights from the Framingham Study. Am Heart J 1985;110:1100–7.

[3] Jacoby RM, Nesto RW. Acute myocardial infarction in the diabetic patient: pathophysiology, clinical course and prognosis. J Am Coll Cardiol 1992;20: 736–44.

[4] Mak KH, Moliterno DJ, Gragner CB, Miller DP, White HD, Wilcox RG, et al. For the GUSTO-I Investigators. Influence of diabetes mellitus on clinical outcome in the thrombolytic era of acute myocardial infarction. J Am Coll Cardiol 1997;30:171–9.

[5] Zuanetti G, Latini R, Maggione AP, Santoro L, Franzosi PG. For the GISSI-2 Investigators. Influence of diabetes on mortality in acute myocardial infarction: data from the GISSI-2 study. J Am Coll Cardiol 1993;22:1788–94.

[6] Cruikshank N. Coronary thrombosis and myocardial infarction, with glycosuria. BMJ 1931;1:618–9.

[7] Sewdarsen M, Jialal I, Vythilingum SS, Govender G, Rajput MC. Stress hyperglycaemia is a predictor of abnormal glucose tolerance in Indian patients with acute myocardial infarction. Diabetes Res 1987;6: 47–9.

[8] Wahab NN, Cowden EA, Pearce NJ, Gardner MJ, Merry H, Cox JL. Is blood glucose an independent predictor of mortality in acute myocardial infarction in the thrombolytic era? J Am Coll Cardiol 2002;40: 1748–54.

[9] Norhammar AM, Ryden L, Malmberg K. Independent risk factor for long-term prognosis after myocardial infarction even in nondiabetic patients. Diabetes Care 1999;22:1827–31.

[10] Capes SE, Hunt D, Malmberg K, Gerstein HC. Stress hyperglycaemia and increased risk of death after myocardial infarction in patients with and

without diabetes: a systematic overview. Lancet 2000;355:773–8.

[11] Malmberg K, Norhammar A, Wedel H, Ryden L. Glycometabolic state at admission: important risk marker of mortality in conventionally treated patients with diabetes mellitus and acute myocardial infarction: long-term results from the diabetes and insulin-glucose infusion in acute myocardial infarction (DIGAMI) study. Circulation 1999;99:2626–32.

[12] Bellodi G, Manicardi V, Malavasi V, et al. Hyperglycemia and prognosis of acute myocardial infarction in patients without diabetes mellitus. Am J Cardiol 1989;64:885–8.

[13] Malmberg K, Ryden L, Hamsten A, Herlitz J, Waldenstrom A, Wedel H. Mortality prediction in diabetic patients with myocardial infarction: experiences from the DIGAMI study. Cardiovasc Res 1997;34:248–53.

[14] Malmberg K, Ryden L, Efendic S, Herrllitz J, Nicol P, Waldenstrom A. A randomized trialglucose infusion followed by subcutaneous insulin treatment in diabetic patients with acute myocardial infarction: effects on one year mortality. J Am Coll Cardiol 1995;26:57–65.

[15] Malmberg K, Ryden L, Hamsten A, Herlitz J, Nicol P, Waldenstrom A, et al. Effects of insulin treatment on cause specific one-year mortality and morbidity in diabetic patients with acute myocardial infarction. Eur Heart J 1996;17:1337–44.

[16] Malmberg K. Prospective randomized study of intensive insulin treatment on long term survival after acute myocardial infarction in patients with diabetes mellitus. BMJ 1997;34:187–220.

[17] Ford ES, Giles WH, Dietz WH. Prevalence of the metabolic syndrome among US adults: findings from the third National Health and Nutritional Examination Survey. JAMA 2002;287:356–9.

[18] Lakka HM, Laaksonen DE, Lakka TA, Niskanen LK, Kumpusalo E, Tuomilehto J, et al. The metabolic syndrome and total and cardiovascular disease mortality in middle-age men. JAMA 2002;288:2709–16.

[19] Norhammar A, Tenerz A, Nilsson G, Hansten A, Efendic S, Ryden L, et al. Glucose metabolism in patients with acute myocardial infarction and no previous diagnosis of diabetes mellitus: a prospective study. Lancet 2002;359:2140–4.

[20] Taubert G, Winkelmann BR, Schleiffer T, Marz W, Winkler R, Gok R, et al. Prevalence, predictors, and consequences of unrecognized diabetes mellitus in 3266 patients scheduled for coronary angiography. Am Heart J 2003;145:285–91.

[21] Kowalska I, Prokop J, Bachorzewska-Galewska H, Telejko B, Kinalskal I, Kochman W, et al. Disturbances of glucose metabolism in men referred for coronary arteriography. Diabetes Care 2001;24: 897–901.

[22] Lopaschuk GD, Stanley WC. Glucose metabolism in the ischemic heart. Circulation 1997;95:313–5.

[23] Taegtmeyer H, McNulty P, Young ME. Adaptation and maladaptation of the heart in diabetes: part I. Circulation 2002;105:1727–33.

[24] Depre C, Vanoverschelde JL, Taegtmeyer H. Glucose for the heart. Circulation 1999;99z:578–88.

[25] Young LH, Renfu Y, Russell R, Hu X, Caplan M, Ren J, et al. Low-flow ischemia leads to translocation of canine heart GLUT-4 and GLUT-1 glucose transporters to the sarcolemma in vivo. Circulation 1997;95:415–22.

[26] Sun D, Nguyen N, DeGrado TR, Schwaiger M, Brosius FC III. Ischemia induces translocation of the insulin-responsive glucose transporter GLUT4 to the plasma membrane of cardiac myocytes. Circulation 1994;89:793–8.

[27] Russell RR III, Yin R, Caplan MJ, Hu X, Ren J, Sholman GI, et al. Additive effects of hyperinsulinemia and ischemia on myocardial GLUT1 and GLUT4 translocation in vivo. Circulation 1998;98: 2180–6.

[28] Sodi-Pallares D, Testelli MR, Fishleder BL, Bisteni A, Medrano GA, et al. Effects of an intravenous infusion of a potassium-insulin-glucose solution on the electrocardiographic signs of myocardial infarction. A preliminary clinical report. Am J Cardiol 1962;9:166–81.

[29] Fath-Ordoubadi F, Beatt KJ. Glucose-insulinpotassium therapy for treatment of acute myocardial infarction: an overview of randomized placebocontrolled trials. Circulation 1997;96:1152–6.

[30] Diaz R, Paolasso EA, Piegas LS, Tajer CD, Moreno MG, Corvalan R, et al. On behalf of the ECLA Collaborative Group. Metabolic modulation of acute myocardial infarction. The ECLA glucoseinsulin-potassium pilot trial. Circulation 1998;98: 2227–34.

[31] Stanley AW Jr, Moraski RE, Russell RO, Rogers WJ, Mantle JA, Kreisberg RA, et al. Effects of glucose-insulin-potassium on myocardial substrate availability and utilization in stable coronary artery disease. Studies on myocardial carbohydrate, lipid and oxygen arterial-coronary sinus differences in patients with coronary artery disease. Am J Cardiol 1975;36:929–37.

[32] Van der Horst ICC, Zijlstra F, van't Hof AW, Doggen CJ, de Boer MJ, Suryapranata H, et al. Glucose-insulin-potassium infusion in patients treated with primary angioplasty for acute myocardial infarction. J Am Coll Cardiol 2003;42:784–91.

[33] Tune JD, Mallet RT, Downey HF. Insulin improves cardiac contractile function and oxygen efficiency during moderate ischemia without compromising myocardial energetics. J Mol Cell Cardiol 1998;30: 2025–35.

[34] Liao R, Jain M, Cui L, D'Agostino J, Aiello F, Luptak I, et al. Cardiac-specific over expression of GLUT1 prevents the development of heart failure attributable to pressure overload in mice. Circulation 2002;106:2125–31.

[35] Jonasen AK, Brar BK, Mjos OD, Sack MN, Latchman DS, Yellon DM. Insulin administered at reoxygenation exerts a cardioprotective effect in myocytes by a possible anti-apoptotic mechanism. J Mol Cell Cardiol 2000;32: 757–64.

[36] Gao F, Gao E, Yue TL, Ohlstein EH, Lopez BL, Christopher TA, et al. Nitric oxide mediates the antiapoptotic effect of in myocardial ischemia-reperfusion: the roles of PI3-kinase, Akt, and endothelial nitric oxide synthase phosphorylation. Circulation 2002;105:1497–502.

[37] Jonassen AK, Aasum E, Riemersma RA, Mjos OD, Larsen TS. Glucose-insulin-potassium reduces infarct size when administered during reperfusion. Cardiovasc Drugs Ther 2000;14:615–23.

[38] Yellon DM, Baxter GF. Protecting the ischaemic and reperfused myocardium in acute myocardial infarction: distinct dream or near reality? Heart 2000; 83:381–7.

[39] Cleveland JC Jr, Meldrum DR, Cain BS, Banerjee A, Harken AH. Oral sulphonylurea hypoglycaemic agents prevent ischemic preconditioning in human myocardium. Two paradoxes revisited. Circulation 1997;96:29–32.

[40] Garratt KN, Brady PA, Hassinger NL, Grill DE, Terzic A, Holmes DR Jr. Sulfonylurea drugs increase early mortality in patients with diabetes mellitus after direct angioplasty for acute myocardial infarction. J Am Coll Cardiol 1999;33: 119–24.

[41] Boord JB, Graber AL, Christman JWS, Powers AC. Practical management of diabetes in critically ill patients. Am J Respir Crit Care Med 2001;164: 1763–7.

[42] Van Den Berghe G, Wouters P, Weekers F, Verwaest C, Bruyninckx F, Schetz M, et al. Intensive insulin therapy in critically ill patients. N Engl J Med 2001;345:1359–67.

[43] Furnary AP, Zerr KJ, Grunkemeier GL, Starr A. Continuous intravenous insulin infusion reduces the incidence of deep sternal wound infection in diabetic patients after cardiac surgical procedures. Ann Thorac Surg 1999;67:352–62.

[44] Lazar HL, Chipkin SR, Fitzgerald CA, Boa Y, Apstein C. Aggressive glucose management optimizes metabolism and reduces morbidity in diabetics coronary bypass patients. Circulation 2002;106: 1972.

[45] Corpus RA, George PB, House JA, Dixon SR, Ajluni SC, Devlin WH, et al. Optimal glycemic control is associated with lower rates of target vessel revascularization in diabetics undergoing elective percutaneous coronary intervention. JACC 2001; 66A:1223–36.

[46] Iribarren C, Karter AJ, Go AS, Ferrara A, Liu JY, Sidney S, et al. Glycemic control and heart failure among adult patients with diabetes. Circulation 2001;103:2668–73.

[47] Conti R. Partial fatty acid oxidation (pFOX) inhibition: a new therapy for chronic stable angina. Clin Cardiol 2003;26:161–2.

[48] Schofield RS, Hill JA. Role of metabolically active drugs in the management of ischemic heart disease. Am J Cardiovasc Drugs 2001;1:23–35.

[49] Schofield RS, Hill JA. The use of ranolazine in cardiovascular disease. Expert Opin Investig Drugs 2002;11(1):117–23.

[50] Yue T, Chen J, Boa W, Narayanan PK, Bril A, Jiang W, et al. In vivo myocardial protection from ischemia/reperfusion injury by the peroxisome proliferator-activated receptor-agonist rosiglitazone. Circulation 2001;104:2588–94.

[51] Shiomi T, Tsutsui H, Hayashidani S, Suematsu N, Ikeuchi M, Wen J, et al. Pioglitazone, a peroxisome proliferator-activated receptor- agonist, attenuates left ventricular remodeling and failure after experimental myocardial infarction. Circulation 2002; 106:3126–32.

[52] Zhu P, Lu L, Xu Y, Schwartz G. Troglitazone improves recovery of left ventricular function after regional ischemia in pigs. Circulation 2000;101: 1165–71.

[53] Parulkar A, Pendergrass ML, Granda-Ayala R, Lee TR, Fonseca VA. Nonhypoglycemic effects of thiazolidinediones. Ann Intern Med 2001;134: 61–71.

[54] Haffner SM, Greenberg AS, Weston WM, Chen H, Williams K, Freed MI. Effect of rosiglitazone treatment on nontraditional markers of cardiovascular disease in patients with type 2 diabetes mellitus. Circulation 2002;106:679–84.

[55] Varo N, Vicent D, Libby P, Nuzzo R, Calle-Pascual AL, Bernal MR, et al. Elevated plasma levels of the atherogenic mediator soluble CD40 ligand in diabetic patients. A novel target of thiazolidinediones. Circulation 2003;107:2664–9.

[56] DeDios ST, Bruemmer D, Dilley RJ, Ivey ME, Jennings GL, Law RE, et al. Inhibitory activity of clinical thiazolidinedione peroxisome proliferator activating receptor- ligands toward internal mammary artery, radial artery, and saphenous vein smooth muscle cell proliferation. Circulation 2003; 107:2548–50.

[57] Choi SH, et al. Diabetes drug, rosiglitazone, reduces in-stent restenosis in diabetics, suggesting anti-inflammatory effects. Presented at the 63rd Session American Diabetes Association Scientific Sessions. June 13–17, 2003. New Orleans.

[58] Minamikawa J, Tanaka S, Yamauchi M, Inoue D, Koshitama H. Potent inhibitory effect of troglitazone on carotid arterial wall thickness in type 2 diabetes. J Clin Endocrinol Metab 1998;83(5):1818–20.

[59] Kirpichnikov D, McFarlane SI, Sowers JR. Metformin: an update. Ann Intern Med 2002;137:25–33.

[60] Mather KJ, Verma S, Anderson TJ. Improved endothelial function with metformin in type 2 diabetes mellitus. J Am Coll Cardiol 2001;37:1344–50.

[61] UK Prospective Diabetes Study (UKPDS) Group. Effect of intensive blood-glucose control with metformin on complications in overweight patients with type 2 diabetes (UKPDS 34). Lancet 1998;352: 854–65.

[62] Mak KH, Topol EJ. Emerging concepts in the management of acute myocardial infarction in patients with diabetes mellitus. J Am Coll Cardiol 2000;35: 563–8.

[63] Poole-Wilson PA, Swedberg K, Cleland JGF, DiLenarda A, Hanrath P, Komajda M, Lubsen J, et al. Comparison of carvedilol and metoprolol on clinical outcomes in patients with chronic heart failure in the Carvedilol or Metoprolol European Trial (COMET): randomised controlled trial. Lancet 2003;362:7–13.

[64] Mathew V, Holmes DR. Outcomes in diabetics undergoing revascularization. J Am Coll Cardiol 2002; 40:423–7.

[65] Libby P, Plutzky J. Diabetic macrovascular disease. The glucose paradox? Circulation 2002;106: 2760–3.

ELSEVIER
SAUNDERS

Cardiol Clin 23 (2005) 119–138

CARDIOLOGY
CLINICS

# Role of Insulin Secretagogues and Insulin Sensitizing Agents in the Prevention of Cardiovascular Disease in Patients who have Diabetes

Ali A. Jawa, MD[a,b], Vivian A. Fonseca, MD[a,b],*

[a]Department of Medicine, Section of Endocrinology, Tulane University Medical Center, SL-53,
1430 Tulane Avenue, New Orleans, LA 70112-2699, USA
[b]Department of Medicine, Veterans Affairs Medical Center, 1601 Perdido Street, New Orleans, LA 70112, USA

Cardiovascular disease is the leading cause of death among patients who have diabetes mellitus. Patients who have diabetes mellitus have a greatly increased relative risk of cardiovascular disease when compared with patients who do not have diabetes mellitus [1]. Furthermore, in patients who have established cardiovascular disease, the rate of subsequent cardiovascular events is significantly higher than in individuals who do not have diabetes mellitus [2] and is associated with greatly increased morbidity and mortality. Epidemiologic studies showed that diabetic patients are more prone to develop complications following cardiovascular events [3]. Moreover, diabetic patients who have ischemic heart disease have a substantially worse outcome after coronary interventional procedures compared with nondiabetic patients [4]. The basis for these differences in outcome remained unclear. In most animal studies, diabetic myocardium demonstrates an enhanced sensitivity to the detrimental effect of ischemia/reperfusion injury and it generally is believed that diabetes mellitus is less tolerant to such injury [3]. Recent advances in invasive cardiology and medical therapy have led to a significant reduction in cardiovascular mortality in nondiabetic men and women; however, the reduction in cardiovascular mortality in men who have diabetes mellitus has been modest and not statistically significant [5], whereas mortality rates increased during a 10-year period in women who had diabetes mellitus.

Diabetes is a complex disease. At least two underlying defects have been postulated in the pathogenesis of this condition. First, β-cell dysfunction and failure that lead to elevated glucose levels result in oxidative stress that causes increased cardiovascular morbidity. Second, insulin resistance, which is associated with endothelial dysfunction, inflammation, and abnormal fibrinolysis contributes to cardiovascular disease [6,7]. Most patients have both defects and the defects frequently are interrelated, in that hyperglycemia itself can lead to insulin resistance and insulin resistance can cause β-cell dysfunction. Fig. 1 illustrates these interactions and outlines a pathway between these defects and cardiovascular disease.

Few long-term studies that compared the effects of secretagogues with sensitizers on cardiovascular outcomes have been conducted. Of particular importance is the United Kingdom Prevention of Diabetes Study (UKPDS), which demonstrated that in obese patients, a weak sensitizer like metformin may be better than a secretagogue in preventing myocardial infarction and cardiovascular mortality.

In the UKPDS, patients who had type 2 diabetes mellitus were randomized to intensive (medication) or conventional (diet) treatment and were observed for approximately 10 years. The group that was assigned to intensive treatment

* Corresponding author. Department of Medicine, Section of Endocrinology, Tulane University Medical Center, SL-53, 1430 Tulane Avenue, New Orleans, LA 70112-2699.

*E-mail address:* vfonseca@tulane.edu (V.A. Fonseca).

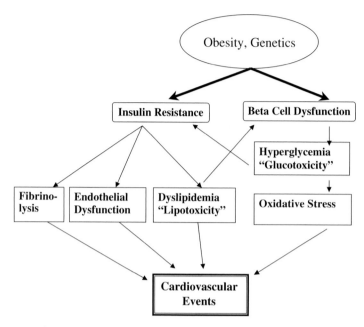

Fig. 1. Pathogenesis of cardiovascular disease in diabetes mellitus.

underwent a subsequent randomization to primary therapy with sulfonylurea or insulin. In addition, obese patients were randomized to metformin or placebo. When compared with conventional therapy, intensive treatment was associated with a decreased risk of predominantly microvascular complications, including a 12% reduction in any diabetes-related end point ($P = 0.03$) and a 25% reduction in all microvascular end points ($P < 0.001$). There was no significant effect on diabetes-related death or on all-cause mortality, however, and there only was a trend toward a small effect ($-16\%$) on the risk of myocardial infarction ($P = 0.05$) [8]. Overall, there were no significant differences between subjects who were treated with sulfonylurea and those who were treated with insulin. Improved glycemic control from sulfonylureas alone is not enough to decrease macrovascular risk. In contrast, obese patients who were randomized to metformin had a reduction in myocardial infarction and cardiovascular mortality. This finding has started a controversial debate about the relative benefits of sensitizers and secretagogues in preventing cardiovascular disease and cardiovascular events.

This article examines the evidence in favor or against choosing treatment with insulin secretagogues or sensitizers as the preferred way to

prevent cardiovascular events. It should be emphasized that most patients eventually will be treated with a combination of therapies; therefore, much of the discussion may not be relevant. Conversely, combination of two sensitizers may have added effects [9,10]. Also, retrospective data suggest that a combination of sulfonylurea and metformin may be associated with increased cardiovascular events [11]. Nevertheless, it is important to recognize the relative value of these different agents as we choose complex therapeutic regimens.

### Effect of glycemic control on cardiovascular disease

Improved blood glucose control decreases the progression of diabetic microvascular disease, but the effect on macrovascular complications is unclear. This is particularly true when older medications are used to treat hyperglycemia. Previously, there was concern that sulfonylureas may increase cardiovascular mortality in patients who have type 2 diabetes mellitus and that high insulin concentrations may enhance atheroma formation. In the UKPDS trial, however, the effects of intensive blood glucose control, with either sulfonylurea or insulin and conventional treatment, on the risk of microvascular and macrovascular complications in patients who had type 2 diabetes mellitus were compared in a randomized, controlled trial [8].

A previous study that was performed in the 1970s, the University Group Diabetes Program (UGDP), concluded that tolbutamide treatment may increase cardiovascular mortality. Criticism of the methodology that was used in the study and the poor overall glycemic control that was achieved reduced the impact of the study. The large (1000 mg) dosage of tolbutamide that was taken in the morning by subjects who were assigned this treatment resulted in a high plasma level for several hours that was followed by a rapid decline due to hepatic clearance.

The Diabetes Mellitus Insulin Glucose Infusion in Acute Myocardial Infarction (DIGAMI) trial is particularly relevant to the impact of glycemic control for cardiology practice. A total of 620 patients were studied; 306 were randomized to treatment with insulin-glucose infusion that was followed by multi-dose subcutaneous insulin for at least 3 months and 314 were randomized to conventional therapy. After 1 year, 57 subjects (18.6%) in the infusion group and 82 subjects (26.1%) in the control group had died (relative mortality reduction 29%, $P = 0.027$). The mortality reduction was particularly evident in patients who had a low cardiovascular risk profile and no previous insulin treatment (3-month mortality rate was 6.5% in the infusion group and 13.5% in the control group [relative reduction 52%, $P = 0.046$]; 1-year mortality rate was 8.6% in the infusion group and 18.0% in the control group [relative reduction 52%, $P = 0.020$]). Insulin-glucose infusion that was followed by a multi-dose insulin regimen improved long-term prognosis in diabetic patients who had acute myocardial infarction [12]. Whether the insulin effect was due to withdrawal of sulfonylurea in DIGAMI is not clear.

*Insulin resistance and cardiovascular disease*

Many of the features of insulin resistance that are present before the onset of hyperglycemia remain operative during the natural history of the diabetes mellitus and contribute greatly to atherosclerosis and associated comorbidities [13,14]. Insulin resistance contributes to the development of atherosclerosis through multiple recognizable risk factors, such as hypertension, dyslipidemia, and hypercoagulability (see Fig. 1) [15].

Insulin resistance and compensatory hyperinsulinemia contribute to hyperglycemia in type 2 diabetes mellitus and may play a pathophysiologic

role in a variety of other metabolic abnormalities, including high levels of plasma triglycerides, low levels of high-density lipoprotein (HDL) cholesterol, hypertension, abnormal fibrinolysis, and coronary heart disease [15,16]. This cluster of abnormalities has been called the insulin resistance syndrome or the metabolic syndrome [17]. The National Cholesterol Education Program Adult Treatment Panel III recently recognized the metabolic syndrome as a secondary therapeutic target for the prevention of cardiovascular diseases [15]. Patients who have the metabolic syndrome meet at least three of the following criteria: triglycerides that are greater than 150 mg/dL, HDL that is less than 40 mg/dL, blood pressure that is greater than 130/85 mm Hg, fasting blood glucose that is greater than 110 mg/dL, and waist circumference that is greater than 40 cm in men or 50 cm in women (Table 1) [15].

## Potential beneficial effects of insulin-sensitizing agents on cardiovascular risk factors

Several epidemiologic studies showed that hyperinsulinemia is an independent risk factor for cardiovascular disease [18]. Correction of insulin resistance clearly is important in the management of type 2 diabetes mellitus and may decrease the risk for cardiovascular disease. In the UKPDS, patients who had type 2 diabetes mellitus and were treated with metformin, which decreases hyperinsulinemia and insulin resistance, had a 30% reduction in cardiovascular disease events and mortality compared with those who received conventional treatment [11]. The thiazolidinediones also improve insulin sensitivity and may exert numerous nonglycemic effects in patients who have type 2 diabetes mellitus [19,20]. Additional clinical trials are being conducted to evaluate whether treatment of diabetes mellitus with agents that reduce insulin resistance, such as the thiazolidinediones, is superior to treatment with agents that stimulate insulin secretion, such as the sulfonylureas.

## Secretagogues

### Sulfonylureas

Sulfonylurea drugs have been available in the United States since 1954. Second-generation sulfonylureas (glyburide, glipizide, and glimepiride) are more potent and probably are safer than first-generation sulfonylureas (chlorpropamide, tolbutamide, acetohexamide, and tolazamide) [21]

Table 1
Effects of the insulin sensitizers on cardiovascular risk factors

| Risk factor | Effect |
| --- | --- |
| Lipids | • Lower triglyceride levels<br>• Increase HDL and LDL cholesterol levels<br>• Decrease LDL cholesterol oxidation and increase LDL cholesterol particle size |
| Coagulation/fibrinolysis | • Reduces PAI-1 and fibrinogen levels |
| Microalbuminuria | • Reduces microalbuminuria |
| Direct vascular effects | • Decrease intima-medial thickness<br>• Lower blood pressure<br>• Increase cardiac output, stroke volume, and peripheral vascular resistance<br>• Induce coronary artery relaxation by decreasing cytosolic calcium<br>• Regulate monocyte/macrophage function in atherosclerotic lesions<br>• Decrease vascular smooth muscle cell migration<br>• Lower calcium influx and attenuate vascular contraction<br>• Reduce carotid intimal inflammation<br>• Decrease renal artery/mesangial cell proliferation |

*Abbreviations:* HDL, high-density lipoprotein; LDL, low-density lipoprotein; PAI, plasminogen activator inhibitor.

Glyburide was associated with increased risk of hypoglycemia; all sulfonylureas cause weight gain and have little impact on other cardiovascular risk factors (Box 1).

*Mechanism of action*

The sulfonylureas bind to the sulfonylurea receptor (SUR) that is found on the surface of pancreatic β cells. This interaction leads to a closure of voltage-dependent ATP-sensitive potassium ($K_{ATP}$) channels and facilitates cell membrane depolarization, calcium entry into the cell, and insulin secretion [26]. Thus, sulfonylureas can lead to insulin release at lower glucose thresholds than normal. They partially reverse the decreased insulin secretion that characterizes type 2 diabetes mellitus [27]; this increases circulating insulin concentrations [23] and lowers blood glucose. The possibility that such agents also may decrease insulin resistance was suggested [22,28]; however, the peripheral effects of sulfonylureas are likely to be secondary to a reduction in "glucotoxicity," rather than a true direct sensitizing effect. With the epidemiologic association between hyperinsulinemia and cardiovascular disease (mainly in nondiabetic patients), some investigators raised concerns that sulfonylureas may increase cardiovascular morbidity [29,30]. Furthermore, sulfonylureas do not have a consistent additional benefit on coexisting conditions, such as elevated lipid levels or blood pressure–major factors that are associated with cardiovascular disease in diabetes mellitus and they also do not have an effect on

---

**Box 1. Advantages and disadvantages of sulfonylureas**

*Advantages*
Generally safe and effective
Cheaper

*Disadvantages*
No effect on insulin resistance
Weight gain, typically from 2 to 5 kg, is problematic in a group of patients who frequently are overweight [7,22–24]
Hypoglycemia that is most likely to affect the elderly, those who have worsening renal function, and those who have irregular meal schedules [7,22,25]. Newer sulfonylurealphonylureas/starlix have less ATP-sensitive potassium binding ($K_{ATP}$), and therefore, cause less hypoglycemia

"nontraditional" risk factors for cardiovascular disease.

An early trial by the UGDP [23], which explored the effectiveness of oral agents versus insulin, found increased cardiovascular mortality in the cohort of patients that was randomized to sulfonylureas. Widespread criticism of the project's methodology placed the validity of its findings in doubt [24]. Nevertheless, concern about cardiovascular risk remains and the package insert for sulfonylureas that is mandated by the US Food and Drug Administration includes a warning about possible cardiovascular risks. In addition, a retrospective analysis of patients who had diabetes mellitus and underwent balloon angioplasty after myocardial infarction reported increased early mortality (odds ratio 2.7 after adjustment for several covariates) in 67 persons who took sulfonylureas and in 118 who used insulin or lifestyle therapy alone [31].

Concern about cardiovascular risk associated with sulfonylureas has been supported by description of a theoretic underlying mechanism—impairment of myocardial ischemic preconditioning. This is a process by which transitory ischemia "conditions" the myocardium in a protective fashion and allows greater tolerance of subsequent ischemia [25,32].

Ischemic preconditioning is a cardioprotective phenomenon in which short periods of myocardial ischemia result in a resistance of the myocardium to a subsequent ischemia [33]. Several studies suggested that preconditioning may result from the activation of $K_{ATP}$ channels [34–36]. Gross and Auchampach [34] were the first investigators to show that preconditioning in dogs is mediated by activation of $K_{ATP}$ channels because it was prevented by glibenclamide. Ischemic preconditioning was shown to be mediated partly by mitochondrial $K_{ATP}$ channels [37]. The opening of these channels may be important in ischemic preconditioning because inhibition of $K_{ATP}$ channels with glibenclamide abolished the cardioprotective effects of ischemic preconditioning in experimental and clinical studies [38,39], and was used to study this phenomenon [40]. Coronary angioplasty is a useful model for clinical study of ischemic preconditioning because it permits adjustment of ischemic time and measurement of metabolic responses to coronary occlusion [25]; however, much of the data are controversial [41–43]. Conflicting evidence largely can be attributed to the use of different species in various studies. Few reports are available about ischemic preconditioning in humans who undergo angioplasty and its effects on cardiovascular events.

This phenomenon was shown experimentally to limit anginal pain, minimize irreversible tissue injury, and protect myocardial function. $K_{ATP}$ channels in myocardial cells have an important role in this process [44,45]. Pharmacologic agents that open $K_{ATP}$ channels have a protective effect similar to that of previous ischemia; agents that close the channels oppose preconditioning by ischemia. Similar (but not identical) $K_{ATP}$ channels also are present in the pancreatic β cell [46,47]. The mechanism of action of sulfonylureas relate to binding to a subunit of the β-cell $K_{ATP}$ channel complex (the SUR) that leads to closure of the channel and stimulation or potentiation of insulin secretion [48,49]. Sulfonylureas also bind to cardiovascular $K_{ATP}$ channels, although less well than to β-cell $K_{ATP}$ channels [47]; presumably, this promotes closure of the channel and opposes ischemic preconditioning. This property of sulfonylureas has the potential to increase cardiovascular risk in patients who have diabetes mellitus.

In addition to animal experiments that support this hypothesis that blockade of ischemic preconditioning may lead to worsening of myocardial ischemia [50,51], several human studies that used glibenclamide tested the clinical relevance of interactions of sulfonylureas with the myocardium. For example, an in vitro study of human atrial tissue compared samples that were obtained during surgery from six diabetic patients who had been taking glibenclamide and one who had been taking glipizide with tissue from a group of four patients who had been taking insulin and six patients who did not have known diabetes mellitus [52]. The atria from patients who were taking a sulfonylurea had less effective protection of contractility during severe hypoxia by previous exposure to hypoxia. Persons who did not have diabetes mellitus were studied during repeated balloon dilation that was done therapeutically for coronary disease. In one study of this kind, 20 patients were randomized to receive a single oral dose of glibenclamide, 10 mg, or placebo just before the procedure [38]. Protection against electrocardiographic changes and pain that resulted during the second balloon dilation in those who were given placebo was abolished by glibenclamide pretreatment. In a second study that accompanied angioplasty, pretreatment with a single intravenous dose of glibenclamide or glimepiride was compared with saline infusion [53].

Electrocardiographic evidence of ischemia was more pronounced during the second period of ischemia after glibenclamide administration compared with glimepiride or placebo. Dipyridamole stress led to more severe worsening of echocardiographically-determined myocardial function when glibenclamide was given.

Thus, blockade of these channels by glibenclamide may worsen myocardial ischemia by preventing ischemic preconditioning. Differential response of myocardial $K_{ATP}$ channels to sulfonylureas was determined by the SUR isoform because multiple regions of SUR contributed to coupling antagonist-occupied sites with the inward rectifier $K^+$ channel-gating machinery [54]. Glimepiride is pharmacologically distinct from glibenclamide because of differences in receptor-binding properties [55]; this could result in a reduced binding to cardiomyocyte $K_{ATP}$ channels as reflected in the lower $K_{ATP}$ channel current inhibition activity [51].

Lee and Chou [56] studied the impact of diabetes mellitus and different sulfonylurea administrations on cardioprotective effects in diabetic patients who were undergoing coronary angioplasty. Myocardial ischemia after coronary angioplasty was evaluated in 20 nondiabetic and 23 diabetic patients who were chronically taking either glibenclamide or glimepiride. Glimepiride significantly lowered the ischemic burden that was assessed by an ST-segment shift, chest pain score, and myocardial lactate extraction ratios compared with glibenclamide in nondiabetic patients; this implied that acute administration of glimepiride did not abolish cardioprotection. In the diabetic group that was treated with glibenclamide, the reduction in the ST-segment shift that was afforded by nicorandil in the first inflation ($-58\%$ versus the first inflation in the glibenclamide group alone) was similar to that afforded by preconditioning ($-59\%$ during the second versus the first inflation). In groups that were treated with glimepiride, the magnitude of attenuated lactate production was less in diabetics than nondiabetics at the second inflation; this suggested that diabetes mellitus plays a role in determining lactate production. These results show that diabetes mellitus and sulfonylureas can act in synergism to inhibit activation of $K_{ATP}$ channels in patients who are undergoing coronary angioplasty. The degree of inhibition that was assessed by metabolic and electrocardiographic parameters was less severe during treatment with glimepiride than with glibenclamide. Restitution of a preconditioning response in patients who are

treated with glimepiride may be the potential beneficial mechanism. Thus, preconditioning leads to protection during subsequent ischemia in nondiabetic patients that is unaffected by glimepiride but impaired by glibenclamide. In the diabetic patients, protection by preconditioning occurred with glimepiride but not with glyburide. In addition, the values for lactate balance suggested that diabetes itself may have impaired preconditioning.

It is possible that whatever effect that glibenclamide has on ischemic preconditioning is counterbalanced by other effects that are beneficial. The most obvious of these is improvement of glycemic control, as in the UKPDS. Another possible protective effect is an antiarrhythmic action of glyburide that seems to occur under certain circumstances [57]. Thus, the effects of glibenclamide on cardiovascular outcomes may remain neutral or favorable despite an undesirable interaction with ischemic preconditioning.

The peak level that is required for adequate duration of action from this short-acting agent might have been high enough to favor significant binding to the lower-affinity myocardial $K_{ATP}$ channel complex and the β-cell channels. Longer-acting sulfonylureas, such as glimepiride, extended-release glipizide, and extended-release gliclazide, lack such prominent peak blood levels, and thus, may be more β-cell specific for pharmacokinetic reasons.

In addition to having effects on the myocardium that set it apart, glibenclamide also may have a greater tendency to cause hypoglycemia than other sulfonylureas [8,58]. As with the myocardial effects, the mechanism of glibenclamide tendency to cause hypoglycemia is not well-defined. Differences in pharmacokinetics, binding properties, and formation and clearance of metabolites may all contribute, particularly in patients who have renal insufficiency. The increased hypoglycemia may pose a problem in patients who are at risk for cardiovascular events. Desouza et al [59] performed continuous glucose monitoring and simultaneous cardiac holter monitoring for ischemia in patients who had type 2 diabetes mellitus that was treated with insulin. Hypoglycemia was more likely to be associated with cardiac ischemia and symptoms than normoglycemia and hyperglycemia and was particularly common in patients who experienced considerable swings in blood glucose. Thus, it may be advisable to avoid drugs that cause hypoglycemia in patients who have established coronary artery disease.

## Nonsulfonylurea secretagogues

This group of drugs stimulates insulin through mechanisms similar to sulfonylureas, but are chemically different and includes repaglinide and nateglinide.

## Mechanism of action

The mechanism of action of the nonsulfonylurea insulin secretagogues (repaglinide [a benzoic acid derivative] and nateglinide [a phenylalanine derivative]) is similar to that of sulfonylureas—interaction with voltage-dependent $K_{ATP}$ channels on β cells. They are distinguished from the sulfonylureas by their short metabolic half-lives, which result in brief episodic stimulation of insulin secretion [60]. There are two important consequences from this difference. First, postprandial glucose excursions are attenuated because of greater insulin secretion immediately after meal ingestion [61]. Second, because less insulin is secreted several hours after the meal, there is decreased risk of hypoglycemia during this late postprandial phase [62]. One agent, nateglinide, has little stimulatory effect on insulin secretion when administered in the fasting state [63]. Thus, nateglinide may enhance meal-stimulated insulin secretion more than do other secretagogues. Efficacy of repaglinide is similar to that of sulfonylureas [64,65], whereas nateglinide seems to be less potent a secretagogue (see Table 1) [66]. Three comparative trials (see Box 1) of repaglinide versus sulfonylurea have been published; each showed equal lowering of glucose levels [67–69]. In single studies, the efficacy of repaglinide was equal to that of metformin [70] but greater than that of troglitazone [71]. In one study, nateglinide was less efficacious than metformin [72].

### Limitations

These drugs have not been assessed for their long-term effectiveness in decreasing microvascular or macrovascular risk. Furthermore, they may cause hypoglycemia and weight gain, which probably are less pronounced than those caused by the sulfonylureas [69]. They require frequent dosing schedule with meals.

## Insulin sensitizers

### Biguanides

Although available internationally for decades, metformin, a biguanide, was not released in the United States until 1995 [73]. An earlier biguanide, phenformin, was removed from the market in the 1970s because of an association with lactic acidosis [74]. In contrast to the sulfonylureas, metformin does not stimulate insulin secretion [75,76]. Metformin is the only biguanide that is available for clinical use (Box 2). Its efficacy as monotherapy and in combination with other agents is well-established [73]. Metformin is the only drug that has been shown to decrease cardiovascular events in patients who have type 2 diabetes mellitus independent of glycemic control [11]. Although metformin has a small effect as a peripheral insulin sensitizer, its main mechanism is inhibiting hepatic gluconeogenesis. Nevertheless, metformin treatment decreases plasma

---

**Box 2. Advantages and disadvantages of metformin**

*Advantages*
Generally safe and effective
Weak insulin sensitizer
Decreases hepatic gluconeogenesis
May cause weight loss which leads to improved insulin resistance
Does not cause hypoglycemia when used as monotherapy
Improves endothelial dysfunction

*Disadvantages*
Requires renal and hepatic function monitoring
May cause significant gastrointestinal side effects in a small subset of patients and sometimes requires discontinuation
Contraindicated in active hepatic, renal, and coronary artery disease

insulin levels and corrects many of the nontraditional risk factors that are associated with the insulin resistance syndrome [77].

*Cardiovascular effects of metformin*

In the UKPDS, treatment with metformin (another drug that decreases hyperinsulinemia and insulin resistance) produced greater reduction in cardiovascular disease events and mortality than sulfonylureas and insulin [8]. The latter drugs decreased blood glucose level to a similar degree as metformin but did not decrease plasma insulin concentrations. This effect may have been mediated through a decrease in insulin resistance, although other effects of metformin, such as improvement in lipid profile, improved fibrinolysis, and prevention of weight gain, may be important [8]. Metformin has a favorable, albeit modest, effect on plasma lipids, particularly in decreasing triglycerides and low-density lipoprotein (LDL) cholesterol; however, it had little, if any, effect on HDL cholesterol levels [78]. Metformin use was associated with decreased plasminogen activator inhibitor (PAI-1) activity which led to improved endothelial dysfunction (see Table 1).

*Thiazolidinediones*

The thiazolidinediones are a relatively new class of compounds for the treatment of type 2 diabetes mellitus (Box 3). Troglitazone became available in the United States in 1997 but was withdrawn from the market in March 2000 because it caused severe idiosyncratic liver injury [79]. The thiazolidinediones have emerged as an important therapeutic drug class in the management of type 2 diabetes mellitus, and their efficacy in lowering plasma glucose is well established [80–

86]. Epidemiologic studies have demonstrated that hyperinsulinemia, a marker for insulin resistance, is an independent risk factor for cardiovascular disease [18]. Correction of insulin resistance may be clinically important in type 2 diabetes mellitus and may decrease risk for cardiovascular disease.

*Mechanism of action*

The glucose-lowering effects of the thiazolidinediones are mediated primarily by decreasing insulin resistance in muscle and fat and, thereby, increasing glucose uptake [19,87]. Thiazolidinediones also increase glucose disposal and reduce hepatic glucose production [88]. The actions of the thiazolidinediones are mediated through binding and activation of the peroxisome proliferator-activated receptor (PPAR)-γ receptor, a nuclear receptor that has a regulatory role in differentiation of cells, particularly adipocytes. This receptor also is expressed in several other tissues, including vascular tissue [89]. In addition, thiazolidinediones decrease plasma free fatty acid concentrations and may improve insulin sensitivity indirectly by this decrease in free fatty acids [90]. Because free fatty acids are involved in lipid metabolism and also have deleterious effects on the vasculature [16], this reduction in plasma free fatty acids may have a beneficial effect on cardiovascular disease.

PPARs are members of the nuclear receptor superfamily and contain common structural elements that include a ligand-binding domain and a DNA-binding domain [91]. Three PPAR family members have been identified thus far, PPAR-γ, PPAR-α, and PPAR-δ (also known as PPAR-β or nuc1). PPAR-γ, a key mediator in metabolic syndromes such as diabetes mellitus and obesity, was identified first as a part of the transcriptional complex that is integral to adipocyte

---

**Box 3. Advantages and disadvantages of thiazolidinediones**

*Advantages*
Potent insulin sensitizer
Cardiovascular benefits
Improves endothelial dysfunction

*Disadvantages*
Requires hepatic function monitoring every 2 months for first year after initiation of therapy
May cause fluid retention
Contraindicated in patients who have New York Heart Association class III and IV congestive heart failure

differentiation. Transient overexpression of PPAR-γ in fibroblasts directs those cells toward an adipocyte-like phenotype [92] that is consistent with high adipose expression of PPAR-γ [93,94]. PPAR-α and PPAR-γ are expressed in the major cellular constituents of the vessel wall (endothelial cell, vascular smooth muscle cell [VSMC], and monocyte/macrophages) as well as in human atherosclerotic lesions [95,96].

The thiazolidinediones have the potential to alter metabolic conditions beyond the management of glycemia [20]. Because the thiazolidinediones target insulin resistance, these agents may improve many of the risk factors that are associated with the insulin resistance syndrome. Although data on the impact of the thiazolidinediones on cardiovascular outcomes are lacking, results of ongoing clinical trials are awaited eagerly [97] and are likely to support the use of these agents in minimizing adverse cardiovascular event. It seems that the thiazolidinediones exert numerous nonglycemic effects that may improve cardiovascular outcomes [19,20].

*Lipid metabolism and oxidation*

Several studies observed the effects of the thiazolidinediones on lipid metabolism [98,99]. Published data indicate that all of the thiazolidinediones increase HDL cholesterol, although only troglitazone and pioglitazone consistently decrease triglycerides [82,100–102]. Pioglitazone and rosiglitazone increase HDL and LDL cholesterol levels. Differences between the thiazolidinediones with respect to their lipid effects may reflect the fact that populations that had different baseline values were studied; a randomized, comparative trial is needed to determine whether a true difference exists.

The effects of the thiazolidinediones on LDL cholesterol are complex. Patients who have type 2 diabetes mellitus (or individuals who are insulin resistant) are more likely than normal individuals to have small, dense, triglyceride-rich LDL cholesterol particles [103] that are highly susceptible to oxidation. Oxidative modification confers atherogenic properties on these small, dense, LDL cholesterol particles [20,104]. This characteristic is a key initial event in the progression of atherosclerosis and the presence of small, dense, LDL is an independent risk factor for cardiovascular disease [105–107]. In some studies, thiazolidinediones increased total cholesterol or LDL cholesterol. Although there is an increase in LDL

cholesterol, this predominantly is in the larger, buoyant particles of LDL cholesterol which may be less atherogenic [90,98,108]. Concomitantly, the small, dense LDL cholesterol particles decreased with thiazolidinedione therapy [98,109]. Winkler et al [110] studied the effect of pioglitazone on LDL subfractions in normolipidemic, nondiabetic patients who had arterial hypertension. They used a monocentric, double-blind, randomized, parallel-group study that compared 45 mg pioglitazone (n = 26) and a placebo (n = 28) that were given once daily for 16 weeks. Fifty-four moderately hypertensive patients (LDL cholesterol, 2.8 mmol/L ± 0.8 mmol/L; HDL cholesterol, 1.1 mmol/L ± 0.3 mmol/L; triglycerides, 1.4 mmol/L (median; range 0.5–7.1 mmol/L) were studied at baseline and on treatment. Pioglitazone reduced dense LDLs by 22% (P = 0.024).

There is evidence to suggest that PPAR-γ may be an important regulator of foam cell gene expression and that oxidized LDL cholesterol regulates macrophage gene expression through activation of PPAR-γ [111]. Chinetti and colleagues [112] demonstrated that activators of PPAR-α and PPAR-γ receptors induce expression of the nuclear receptor liver x receptor–α and ATP-binding cassette subfamily–1 promoter genes, which are involved in the pathway that activates apolipoprotein AI–mediated cholesterol efflux from macrophages and macrophage-derived foam cells. Furthermore, PPAR-γ promotes the uptake of oxidized LDL cholesterol by macrophages [113].

*Blood pressure*

If insulin resistance causes hypertension, then improving insulin sensitivity should have the potential to lower blood pressure. The effects of thiazolidinediones on blood pressure have been examined in several different experimental and clinical settings. A study of 24 nondiabetic, hypertensive patients who were treated with rosiglitazone demonstrated that rosiglitazone treatment added to the patient's usual antihypertensive medication resulted in a decline in systolic and diastolic blood pressure and improved insulin resistance [114]. Ogihara and associates [115] demonstrated significant reduction in blood pressure in hypertensive subjects who had type 2 diabetes mellitus and were treated with troglitazone. In another study of 203 patients who had type 2 diabetes mellitus, treatment with rosiglitazone significantly reduced ambulatory blood pressure [116]. Scherbaum and associates [117] also reported decreases in systolic blood pressure by pioglitazone in normotensive and hypertensive patients who had diabetes mellitus. Similar results were seen in nonhypertensive patients who had type 2 diabetes mellitus [82] and nondiabetic, obese persons [83,118].

Raji et al [114] examined the effect of rosiglitazone on insulin resistance and blood pressure in patients who had essential hypertension. There were significant decreases in mean 24-hour systolic blood pressure; the decline in systolic blood pressure correlated with the improvement in insulin sensitivity. Rosiglitazone treatment of nondiabetic hypertensive patients improves insulin sensitivity, reduces systolic and diastolic blood pressure, and induces favorable changes in markers of cardiovascular risk.

A potential mechanism for thiazolidinedione-mediated decreases in blood pressure may be improved insulin sensitivity, which promotes insulin-mediated vasodilatation. Alternative hypotheses for the decrease in blood pressure include inhibition of intracellular calcium and myocyte contractility [119,120] and endothelin-1 expression and secretion. Pioglitazone inhibited renal artery proliferation in animal models [121,122] which generated reductions in blood pressure.

*Endothelial function, vascular reactivity, and vascular wall abnormalities*

Vascular endothelium is involved in the regulation of vascular tone, vessel permeability, and angiogenesis. Various paracrine vasodilatory and vasoconstrictor factors, most notably nitric oxide and endothelin-1, determine vascular tone [80,123]. The endothelium plays a vital role in the maintenance of blood fluidity, vascular wall tone, and permeability. Endothelial dysfunction is central to many vascular diseases, including atherosclerosis and diabetic microangiopathy. Endothelial function is disturbed by many of the individual features of the insulin resistance syndrome, including hypertension, dyslipidemia, and hyperglycemia [124].

In insulin-resistant, obese subjects and patients who have type 2 diabetes mellitus, this vasodilatory effect of insulin is decreased—an abnormality that might be attributable to impairment in the ability of the endothelium to produce nitric oxide or to enhanced inactivation of nitric oxide [122]. In addition, the action of endothelium-derived nitric oxide is impaired in patients who have atherosclerosis and insulin resistance. This impairment has been attributed, in part, to increased vascular oxidative stress. Thiazolidinediones improve endothelium-derived nitric oxide production and action, and hence, may be a potential agent in the treatment of patients who have coronary artery disease [125]. An antioxidant effect of the thiazolidinediones also inhibits the expression of adhesion molecules by the endothelial cells. Thiazolidinediones inhibit the expression of proinflammatory genes (nuclear factor KB [NFκB]-regulated genes) and suppresses factors that are responsible for plaque rupture and thrombosis (ie, early growth response transcription factor–1 and tissue factor), which could contribute to an antiatherogenic effect [126].

Avena and colleagues [127] demonstrated normalization of impaired brachial artery flow–mediated dilatation in troglitazone-treated human subjects who had peripheral vascular disease. Improvement of vascular reactivity in obese, nondiabetic patients after treatment with rosiglitazone also was reported [128]. The thiazolidinediones act on the endothelium by way of various mechanisms, namely their action on the nitric oxide synthesis; modulation of the nuclear receptor, PPAR-γ; and effects on various cytokines, including adhesion molecules, that are involved in the atherosclerotic process [129–131]. Recently, metformin was shown to improve endothelial function [100]. Because the biguanides do not stimulate PPARs, other mechanisms are likely to be involved in the pathogenesis of endothelial dysfunction in insulin resistance.

The thiazolidinediones also may prevent the progression of atherosclerosis by inhibiting monocyte chemoattractant protein (MCP)-1 expression in endothelial cells. In addition to attenuated response to tumor necrosis factor (TNF)-α, other mediators of inflammation also are suppressed. Anti-inflammatory properties and antioxidant effects were observed in patients who had type 2 diabetes mellitus and were treated with thiazolidinediones; hence, these agents may be of benefit at the vascular level [125,129–132]. One study that evaluated troglitazone showed a profound reduction in the levels of NFκB, a molecule that induces inflammatory cytokines, such as TNF-α, MCP-1, adhesion molecules (soluble intercellular adhesion molecule–1), and reactive oxygen species. Thus, thiazolidinediones exert anti-inflammatory actions that may contribute to their putative antiatherosclerotic effects [133].

PPAR-$\gamma$ ligands counter the effects of various inflammatory cytokines that are released after the endothelial injury. These agents also inhibit VSMC proliferation, down-regulate endothelial cell growth factor receptors, and suppress the movement of various other cells through inhibition of vascular cell adhesion molecule (VCAM)-1, intercellular adhesion molecule (ICAM)-1, and MCP-1. A recent animal study demonstrated that pioglitazone had vasculoprotective effects in acute and chronic vascular injury [131]. Similarly, in a rat model, rosiglitazone reduced myocardial infarction and postischemic injury and improved aortic flow following reperfusion [134,135].

B-mode ultrasound is a noninvasive method for evaluating carotid intimal-medial complex thickness, which is an indicator for early atherosclerosis and is associated with insulin resistance [136,137]. This measurement may serve as a surrogate marker for atherosclerotic events because patients who have increased intimal-medial complex thickness have a higher rate of cardiovascular events over time. Treatment with troglitazone significantly decreases intima-medial thickness in patients who had type 2 diabetes mellitus [137]. Koshiyama and associates [138] recently reported a significant decrease in the intima-medial thickness in patients who had type 2 diabetes mellitus and were treated with pioglitazone. It is possible that the effects of the thiazolidinediones are direct cellular effects on the atherosclerotic process that are not linked to their effects on insulin resistance.

In acute coronary events, exposure of the highly thrombogenic lipid core to circulating coagulation factors can lead to a progressive cascade that results in occlusion of the vessel. Matrix metalloproteinases (MMPs) that are produced by monocyte-derived macrophages and vascular smooth muscle cells contribute to this process by causing plaque rupture, and thus, exposure of the lipid core. Troglitazone and rosiglitazone inhibited the expression and functional activity of MMP-9 in human monocyte–derived macrophages and human VSMC [96,139,140]. Patients with Type 2 diabetes are disproportionately affected by cardiovascular disease, and cardiovascular events are a major cause for morbidity and mortality in this population [141]. Following cardiovascular interventions such as balloon angioplasty, patients with diabetes appear to have a higher rate of restenosis [142]. Several recent human trials have demonstrated beneficial effects of thiazolidenediones in decreasing restenosis

following angioplasty. Choi et al [143] have recently demonstrated that patients having a coronary stent implant who were randomized to receive rosiglitazone had a significant reduction in restenosis as well as artery diameter reduction compared to a control group who received equal glucose lowering therapy with other agents (Fig. 2). Similarly, pioglitazone has been demonstrated to reduce neointimal tissue proliferation after coronary stent implantation in patients with type 2 diabetes mellitus [144]. Although small clinical studies discussed above are interesting, large multicenter studies are needed to confirm these findings before they can be translated into clinical practice [141].

In summary, thiazolidinediones improve endothelial nitric oxide synthesis, counter the effects of hyperinsulinemia-induced resistance, suppress various mediators of inflammation that are involved in atherosclerosis, and inhibit injury-induced VSMC migration; thereby, they potentially prevent restenosis and further occlusion.

*Fibrinolysis, coagulation, and inflammation*

Decreased fibrinolytic activity, in association with elevated plasma PAI-1, is associated with an

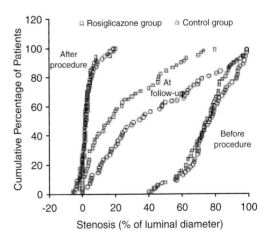

Fig. 2. Cumulative distribution curves for percent stenosis of the luminal diameter in the rosiglitazone and central groups. The distributions were similar at baseline and immediately after stent implantation. At 6 months the mean degree of stenosis in the rosiglitazone group was significantly lower than in the control group. (*From* Choi D, Kim SK, Choi SH. Preventative effects of rosiglitazone on restenosis after coronary stent implantation in patients with type 2 diabetes. Diabetes Care 2004;27:2654–60; with permission.)

increased risk of atherosclerosis and cardiovascular disease [145,146]. PAI-1 is the primary inhibitor of endogenous tissue plasminogen activator and is elevated in patients who have diabetes mellitus and in insulin-resistant nondiabetic individuals. Increased PAI-1 levels are now recognized to be an integral part of the insulin resistance syndrome and correlate significantly with plasma insulin. Insulin infusion during infarction and postinfarction periods (which is known to improve outcomes) decreased plasma PAI-1 levels [147]. Immunohistochemical analysis of the coronary lesions from patients who had coronary artery disease demonstrated an imbalance of the local fibrinolytic system with increased coronary artery tissue PAI-1 levels in patients who had type 2 diabetes mellitus [148]. Impaired fibrinolysis also is noted in other insulin-resistant states, such as the polycystic ovary syndrome [138]. Fonseca and colleagues [149] demonstrated a decrease in plasma PAI-1 levels in patients who had diabetes mellitus who treated with a thiazolidinedione. This observation was confirmed in several studies [124,150]. The postulated mechanism for the effect of the thiazolidinediones is by way of the activation of PPAR-$\gamma$ and subsequent suppression of PAI-1.

In vitro studies with troglitazone demonstrated direct effect on the vessel wall that led to a decreased synthesis of PAI-1 and indirect effects on hepatic synthesis as a result of the attenuation of hyperinsulinemia [151]. Pioglitazone had a similar effect [132]. Treatment with rosiglitazone also decreased PAI-1 levels [152]. Therefore, PAI-1 reduction may well be a class effect of the insulin sensitizers. Although increases in PAI-1 levels are associated with an increased risk of myocardial infarction, no study demonstrated a diminution of this risk with reduction in plasma PAI-1 levels. Consequently, clinical trials are necessary to demonstrate such a benefit.

Like elevated PAI-1, increases in plasma concentrations of markers of inflammation, such as C-reactive protein (CRP), are associated with the insulin resistance syndrome and cardiovascular disease [153]. Fuell and colleagues [154] reported reductions in the proinflammatory markers, interleukin-6, CRP, and white blood cells, in patients who had type 2 diabetes mellitus that was treated with rosiglitazone. Haffner and colleagues [155] reported a reduction in levels of MMP-9 and CRP in patients who had type 2 diabetes mellitus and were treated with rosiglitazone. These effects may be related to the decrease in insulin resistance

and may have beneficial consequences for long-term cardiovascular risk.

Mohanty et al [156] treated 11 nondiabetic obese subjects and 11 obese diabetic subjects with 4 mg of rosiglitazone daily for a period of 6 weeks. Blood glucose concentration changed significantly at 6 weeks only in the obese diabetic subjects after rosiglitazone treatment for 6 weeks, whereas insulin concentration decreased significantly at 6 weeks in both groups. Rosiglitazone treatment led to a significant reduction in NF$\kappa$B-binding activity in mononuclear cells, plasma MCP-1, TNF-$\alpha$, soluble MCP-1, CRP, and serum amyloid A were also lowered, particularly in the obese patients. Thus, rosiglitazone, a selective PPAR-$\gamma$ agonist, exerts an antiinflammatory effect at the cellular and molecular level, and in plasma.

### Albuminuria

Urinary microalbuminuria is monitored routinely in clinical practice and is recognized as a marker of cardiovascular disease and diabetic nephropathy [157,158]. Current methods of reducing microalbuminuria include strict glycemic control and the use of angiotensin-converting enzyme inhibitors. Imano and colleagues [157] showed reductions in urinary microalbumin: creatinine ratio during a 12-week clinical trial when troglitazone was compared with metformin. Similar effects were noted with rosiglitazone. [116,159]. In a 52-week, open trial of patients who had type 2 diabetes mellitus who were given either rosiglitazone or glyburide, patients who were treated with rosiglitazone had a significant reduction in urinary albumin:creatinine ratio compared with baseline [116]. Laboratory work revealed that PPAR-$\gamma$ receptors are expressed in mesangial cells of animal models and inhibit mesangial cell proliferation and angiotensin II–induced PAI-1 expression [160]. Consequently, thiazolidinedione therapy may represent an alternate method for reducing proteinuria and subsequent nephropathy.

### Body weight

Clinical trials suggest that thiazolidinediones may increase body weight; however, the weight gain is accompanied by improvement in glycemic control and also may be secondary to fluid retention [161–163]. Stimulation of adipogenesis through PPAR-$\gamma$ is another potential mechanism for weight gain [164]. This effect is site-specific; weight gain occurs from an increase in subcutaneous fat with a concomitant decrease in visceral fat content (ie, fat redistribution) [165–167]. The clinical significance of increased body weight with the thiazolidinediones is unclear. Weight gain usually increases insulin resistance, which, in turn, increases glucose; however, thiazolidinediones clearly decrease insulin resistance and glucose despite mild weight gain.

Thus, other mechanisms must be involved in the weight/insulin resistance relationship. For instance, increased intra-abdominal fat is associated with increased insulin resistance [168,169]. The redistribution of body fat that is mediated by the thiazolidinediones may be important; studies support this hypothesis. Kelly and associates [166] demonstrated that treatment with troglitazone in human subjects who had type 2 diabetes mellitus decreased intra-abdominal fat mass but did not affect total body fat or weight. Similar effects were observed in patients who had type 2 diabetes mellitus who were treated with rosiglitazone or pioglitazone [170,171]. Thus, the thiazolidinediones may reduce fat accumulation in the visceral abdominal cavity by improving insulin sensitivity.

### Choosing treatment

Type 2 diabetes mellitus is one of the major risk factors for coronary artery disease; the optimal treatment of established coronary artery disease (CAD) in these patients remains controversial. The Bypass Angioplasty Revascularization Investigation (BARI) compared the outcome of percutaneous transluminal coronary angioplasty (PTCA) with coronary artery bypass graft (CABG) surgery [172]; no significant difference between PTCA and CABG was found. In the diabetes subgroup, however, mortality was higher in patients who underwent PTCA compared with CABG (34.5% versus 19.4%, $P = 0.0024$, relative risk, 1.87) [173]. A 7-year follow-up showed a statistically significant survival advantage for patients who received CABG compared with those who received PTCA [174]. The theoretic potential of sulfonylureas to interfere with ischemic preconditioning adds to the controversy that surrounds the use of invasive interventions in diabetics [52]. This may result in greater tissue loss in patients who are treated with these drugs, although recent data suggest that some of the newer sulfonylureas may have a lower tendency to cause this problem. It also is important to recognize that metformin should be discontinued before such procedures.

A new study, the BARI 2 Diabetes (BARI 2D), is being performed in patients who have type 2 diabetes mellitus and documented CAD [175]. The aim of this study is to compare treatment efficacy between initial elective revascularization, either surgical or catheter-based, combined with aggressive medical therapy and aggressive medical therapy alone. Also, this trial compares 5-year mortality in a strategy of hyperglycemia management with insulin sensitizers versus insulin secretagogues. The prevalence of diabetes mellitus in the United States is enormous and is increasing rapidly. Patients who have diabetes mellitus respond less favorably to percutaneous coronary interventions and surgery compared with nondiabetic patients. These considerations led to the initiation of the BARI 2D trial. It is designed to determine whether treatment that is targeted to attenuate insulin resistance can arrest or retard progression of CAD compared with treatment that is targeted to the same level of glycemic control with an insulin-providing approach. It also is designed to determine whether early revascularization reduces mortality and morbidity in patients who have type 2 diabetes mellitus whose cardiac symptoms are mild and stable.

### Summary

In the absence of clinical trial evidence to compare the secretagogues with sensitizers, it is difficult to make recommendations about which class of drug is more important to prescribe for the prevention of cardiovascular disease in diabetes mellitus. Epidemiologic data supports insulin resistance as a major factor in cardiovascular disease through a variety of mechanisms. Because sensitizers improve insulin sensitivity and correct many of the vascular abnormalities that are associated with insulin resistance, it is tempting to suggest that they may be superior for this purpose. Conversely, meeting the goals that are recommended for glycemia also are important and achieving them may not be always possible with sensitizers, particularly in the later stages of the disease when insulin levels are not high, despite insulin resistance. In such situations, combination therapy may be needed with both types of drugs [176–179]. No data are available on the cardiovascular effects of such combinations; some retrospective data suggest a possibility of

increased events with the combination of sulfonylureas and metformin [11]. Thus, further prospective studies in this area are necessary.

## References

[1] Kannel WB, McGee DL. Diabetes and cardiovascular disease. The Framingham study. JAMA
1979;241(19):2035–8.

[2] Haffner SM. Management of dyslipidemia in adults
with diabetes. Diabetes Care 1998;21(1):160–78.

[3] Stone PH, Muller JE, Hartwell T, York BJ, Rutherford JD, Parker CB, et al. The effect of diabetes
mellitus on prognosis and serial left ventricular
function after acute myocardial infarction: contri-
bution of both coronary disease and diastolic left
ventricular dysfunction to the adverse prognosis.
The MILIS Study Group. J Am Coll Cardiol
1989;14(1):49–57.

[4] Stein B, Weintraub WS, Gebhart SP, Cohen-Bernstein CL, Grosswald R, Liberman HA, et al. Influence of diabetes mellitus on early and late
outcome after percutaneous transluminal coronary
angioplasty. Circulation 1995;91(4):979–89.

[5] Gu K, Cowie CC, Harris MI. Diabetes and decline
in heart disease mortality in US adults. JAMA
1999;281(14):1291–7.

[6] Lillioja S, Mott DM, Spraul M, Ferraro R, Foley
JE, Ravussin E, et al. Insulin resistance and
insulin secretory dysfunction as precursors of
non-insulin-dependent diabetes mellitus. Prospective studies of Pima Indians. N Engl J Med 1993;
329(27):1988–92.

[7] Ferrannini E. Insulin resistance versus insulin deficiency in non-insulin-dependent diabetes mellitus:
problems and prospects. Endocr Rev 1998;19(4):
477–90.

[8] UK Prospective Diabetes Study (UKPDS) Group.
Intensive blood-glucose control with sulphonylureas or insulin compared with conventional treatment and risk of complications in patients with type
2 diabetes (UKPDS 33). Lancet 1998;352(9131):
837–53.

[9] Einhorn D, Rendell M, Rosenzweig J, Egan JW,
Mathisen AL, Schneider RL. Pioglitazone hydro-
chloride in combination with metformin in the
treatment of type 2 diabetes mellitus: a randomized, placebo-controlled study. The Pioglitazone
027 Study Group. Clin Ther 2000;22(12):
1395–409.

[10] Fonseca V, Rosenstock J, Patwardhan R, Salzman
A. Effect of metformin and rosiglitazone combination therapy in patients with type 2 diabetes mellitus: a randomized controlled trial. JAMA 2000;
283(13):1695–702.

[11] UK Prospective Diabetes Study (UKPDS) Group.
Effect of intensive blood-glucose control with metformin on complications in overweight patients

with type 2 diabetes (UKPDS 34). Lancet 1998;
352(9131):854–65.

[12] Malmberg K, Ryden L, Efendic S, Herlitz J, Nicol
P, Waldenstrom A, et al. Randomized trial of insulin-glucose infusion followed by subcutaneous
insulin treatment in diabetic patients with acute
myocardial infarction (DIGAMI study): effects
on mortality at 1 year. J Am Coll Cardiol 1995;
26(1):57–65.

[13] Brunzell JD, Hokanson JE. Dyslipidemia of central
obesity and insulin resistance. Diabetes Care 1999;
22(Suppl 3):C10–3.

[14] Ginsberg HN, Huang LS. The insulin resistance
syndrome: impact on lipoprotein metabolism and
atherothrombosis. J Cardiovasc Risk 2000;7(5):
325–31.

[15] Expert Panel on Detection, Evaluation, And Treatment of High Blood Cholesterol In Adults (Adult
Treatment Panel III). Executive Summary of The
Third Report of The National Cholesterol Education Program (NCEP). JAMA 2001;285(19):
2486–97.

[16] Steinberg HO, Paradisi G, Hook G, Crowder K,
Cronin J, Baron AD. Free fatty acid elevation
impairs insulin-mediated vasodilation and nitric
oxide production. Diabetes 2000;49(7):1231–8.

[17] Reaven GM, Lithell H, Landsberg L. Hypertension
and associated metabolic abnormalities—the role
of insulin resistance and the sympathoadrenal
system. N Engl J Med 1996;334(6):374–81.

[18] Despres JP, Lamarche B, Mauriege P, Cantin B,
Dagenais GR, Moorjani S, et al. Hyperinsulinemia
as an independent risk factor for ischemic heart
disease. N Engl J Med 1996;334(15):952–7.

[19] Martens FM, Visseren FL, Lemay J, de Koning EJ,
Rabelink TJ. Metabolic and additional vascular
effects of thiazolidinediones. Drugs 2002;62(10):
1463–80.

[20] Parulkar AA, Pendergrass ML, Granda-Ayala R,
Lee TR, Fonseca VA. Nonhypoglycemic effects of
thiazolidinediones. Ann Intern Med 2001;134(1):
61–71.

[21] Cohen KL, Harris S. Efficacy of glyburide in
diabetics poorly controlled on first-generation
oral hypoglycemics. Diabetes Care 1987;10(5):
555–7.

[22] Kolterman OG, Prince MJ, Olefsky JM. Insulin resistance in noninsulin-dependent diabetes mellitus:
impact of sulfonylurea agents in vivo and in vitro.
Am J Med 1983;74(1A):82–101.

[23] Goldner MG, Knatterud GL, Prout TE. Effects of
hypoglycemic agents on vascular complications in
patients with adult-onset diabetes. 3. Clinical implications of UGDP results. JAMA 1971;218(9):
1400–10.

[24] Kilo C, Miller JP, Williamson JR. The crux of the
UGDP. Spurious results and biologically inappro-
priate data analysis. Diabetologia 1980;18(3):
179–85.

[25] Deutsch E, Berger M, Kussmaul WG, Hirshfeld JW Jr, Herrmann HC, Laskey WK. Adaptation to ischemia during percutaneous transluminal coronary angioplasty. Clinical, hemodynamic, and metabolic features. Circulation 1990;82(6): 2044–51.

[26] Zimmerman BR. Sulfonylureas. Endocrinol Metab Clin North Am 1997;26(3):511–22.

[27] Doar JW, Thompson ME, Wilde CE, Sewell PF. Diet and oral antidiabetic drugs and plasma sugar and insulin levels in patients with maturity-onset diabetes mellitus. BMJ 1976;1(6008):498–500.

[28] Simonson DC, Ferrannini E, Bevilacqua S, Smith D, Barrett E, Carlson R, et al. Mechanism of improvement in glucose metabolism after chronic glyburide therapy. Diabetes 1984;33(9):838–45.

[29] Garratt KN, Brady PA, Hassinger NL, Grill DE, Terzic A, Holmes DR Jr. Sulfonylurea drugs increase early mortality in patients with diabetes mellitus after direct angioplasty for acute myocardial infarction. J Am Coll Cardiol 1999;33(1):119–24.

[30] Henry RR. Type 2 diabetes care: the role of insulin-sensitizing agents and practical implications for cardiovascular disease prevention. Am J Med 1998;105(1A):20S–6S.

[31] Garratt KN, Brady PA, Hassinger NL, Grill DE, Terzic A, Holmes DR Jr. Sulfonylurea drugs increase early mortality in patients with diabetes mellitus after direct angioplasty for acute myocardial infarction. J Am Coll Cardiol 1999;33(1):119–24.

[32] Kloner RA, Yellon D. Does ischemic preconditioning occur in patients? [abstract]. J Am Coll Cardiol 1994;24(4):1133–42.

[33] Murry CE, Jennings RB, Reimer KA. Preconditioning with ischemia: a delay of lethal cell injury in ischemic myocardium. Circulation 1986;74(5): 1124–36.

[34] Gross GJ, Auchampach JA. Blockade of ATP-sensitive potassium channels prevents myocardial preconditioning in dogs. Circ Res 1992;70(2):223–33.

[35] Grover GJ, Sleph PG, Dzwonczyk S. Role of myocardial ATP-sensitive potassium channels in mediating preconditioning in the dog heart and their possible interaction with adenosine A1-receptors. Circulation 1992;86(4):1310–6.

[36] Cole WC, McPherson CD, Sontag D. ATP-regulated K$^+$ channels protect the myocardium against ischemia/reperfusion damage. Circ Res 1991;69(3):571–81.

[37] Lee TM, Su SF, Tsai CC, Lee YT, Tsai CH. Cardioprotective effects of 17 beta-estradiol produced by activation of mitochondrial ATP-sensitive K(+)Channels in canine hearts. J Mol Cell Cardiol 2000;32(7):1147–58.

[38] Tomai F, Crea F, Gaspardone A, Versaci F, De Paulis R, Penta dP, et al. Ischemic preconditioning during coronary angioplasty is prevented by glibenclamide, a selective ATP-sensitive K$^+$ channel blocker. Circulation 1994;90(2):700–5.

[39] Qian YZ, Levasseur JE, Yoshida K, Kukreja RC. KATP channels in rat heart: blockade of ischemic and acetylcholine-mediated preconditioning by glibenclamide. Am J Physiol 1996;271(1 Pt 2): H23–8.

[40] Sato T, Sasaki N, O'Rourke B, Marban E. Nicorandil, a potent cardioprotective agent, acts by opening mitochondrial ATP-dependent potassium channels. J Am Coll Cardiol 2000;35(2):514–8.

[41] Fenton RA, Dickson EW, Meyer TE, Dobson JG Jr. Aging reduces the cardioprotective effect of ischemic preconditioning in the rat heart. J Mol Cell Cardiol 2000;32(7):1371–5.

[42] Abete P, Ferrara N, Cioppa A, Ferrara P, Bianco S, Calabrese C, et al. Preconditioning does not prevent postischemic dysfunction in aging heart. J Am Coll Cardiol 1996;27(7):1777–86.

[43] Burns PG, Krunkenkamp IB, Calderone CA, Kirvaitis RJ, Gaudette GR, Levitsky S. Is the preconditioning response conserved in senescent myocardium? Ann Thorac Surg 1996;61(3):925–9.

[44] O'Rourke B. Myocardial K(ATP) channels in preconditioning. Circ Res 2000;87(10):845–55.

[45] Terzic A, Jahangir A, Kurachi Y. Cardiac ATP-sensitive K$^+$ channels: regulation by intracellular nucleotides and K$^+$ channel-opening drugs. Am J Physiol 1995;269(3 Pt 1):C525–45.

[46] Aguilar-Bryan L, Clement JP, Gonzalez G, Kunjilwar K, Babenko A, Bryan J. Toward understanding the assembly and structure of KATP channels. Physiol Rev 1998;78(1):227–45.

[47] Lazdunski M. Ion channel effects of antidiabetic sulfonylureas. Horm Metab Res 1996;28(9):488–95.

[48] Kramer W, Muller G, Geisen K. Characterization of the molecular mode of action of the sulfonylurea, glimepiride, at beta-cells. Horm Metab Res 1996;28(9):464–8.

[49] Ashcroft FM. Mechanisms of the glycaemic effects of sulfonylureas. Horm Metab Res 1996;28(9): 456–63.

[50] Mocanu MM, Maddock HL, Baxter GF, Lawrence CL, Standen NB, Yellon DM. Glimepiride, a novel sulfonylurea, does not abolish myocardial protection afforded by either ischemic preconditioning or diazoxide. Circulation 2001;103(25): 3111–6.

[51] Geisen K, Vegh A, Krause E, Papp JG. Cardiovascular effects of conventional sulfonylureas and glimepiride. Horm Metab Res 1996;28(9):496–507.

[52] Cleveland JC Jr, Meldrum DR, Cain BS, Banerjee A, Harken AH. Oral sulfonylurea hypoglycemic agents prevent ischemic preconditioning in human myocardium. Two paradoxes revisited. Circulation 1997;96(1):29–32.

[53] Klepzig H, Kober G, Matter C, Luus H, Schneider H, Boedeker KH, et al. Sulfonylureas and ischaemic preconditioning; a double-blind, placebo-controlled evaluation of glimepiride and glibenclamide. Eur Heart J 1999;20(6):439–46.

[54] Babenko AP, Bryan J. A conserved inhibitory and differential stimulatory action of nucleotides on K(IR)6.0/SUR complexes is essential for excitation-metabolism coupling by K(ATP) channels. J Biol Chem 2001;276(52):49083–92.

[55] Muller G, Hartz D, Punter J, Okonomopulos R, Kramer W. Differential interaction of glimepiride and glibenclamide with the beta-cell sulfonylurea receptor. I. Binding characteristics. Biochim Biophys Acta 1994;1191(2):267–77.

[56] Lee TM, Chou TF. Impairment of myocardial protection in type 2 diabetic patients. J Clin Endocrinol Metab 2003;88(2):531–7.

[57] Tosaki A, Szerdahelyi P, Engelman RM, Das DK. Potassium channel openers and blockers: do they possess proarrhythmic or antiarrhythmic activity in ischemic and reperfused rat hearts? J Pharmacol Exp Ther 1993;267(3):1355–62.

[58] Holstein A, Plaschke A, Egberts EH. Lower incidence of severe hypoglycaemia in patients with type 2 diabetes treated with glimepiride versus glibenclamide. Diabetes Metab Res Rev 2001; 17(6):467–73.

[59] Desouza C, Salazar H, Cheong B, Murgo J, Fonseca V. Association of hypoglycemia and cardiac ischemia: a study based on continuous monitoring. Diabetes Care 2003;26(5):1485–9.

[60] Perfetti R, Ahmad A. Novel sulfonylurea and non-sulfonylurea drugs to promote the secretion of insulin. Trends Endocrinol Metab 2000;11(6): 218–23.

[61] Hirschberg Y, Karara AH, Pietri AO, McLeod JF. Improved control of mealtime glucose excursions with coadministration of nateglinide and metformin. Diabetes Care 2000;23(3):349–53.

[62] Nattrass M, Lauritzen T. Review of prandial glucose regulation with repaglinide: a solution to the problem of hypoglycaemia in the treatment of type 2 diabetes? Int J Obes Relat Metab Disord 2000; 24(Suppl 3):S21–31.

[63] Keilson L, Mather S, Walter YH, Subramanian S, McLeod JF. Synergistic effects of nateglinide and meal administration on insulin secretion in patients with type 2 diabetes mellitus. J Clin Endocrinol Metab 2000;85(3):1081–6.

[64] Goldberg RB, Einhorn D, Lucas CP, Rendell MS, Damsbo P, Huang WC, et al. A randomized placebo-controlled trial of repaglinide in the treatment of type 2 diabetes. Diabetes Care 1998; 21(11):1897–903.

[65] Jovanovic L, Dailey G III, Huang WC, Strange P, Goldstein BJ Repaglinide in type 2 diabetes: a 24-week, fixed-dose efficacy and safety study. J Clin Pharmacol 2000;40(1):49–57.

[66] Hanefeld M, Bouter KP, Dickinson S, Guitard C. Rapid and short-acting mealtime insulin secretion with nateglinide controls both prandial and mean glycemia. Diabetes Care 2000;23(2): 202–7.

[67] Wolffenbuttel BH, Landgraf R. A 1-year multicenter randomized double-blind comparison of repaglinide and glyburide for the treatment of type 2 diabetes. Dutch and German Repaglinide Study Group. Diabetes Care 1999;22(3):463–7.

[68] Landgraf R, Bilo HJ, Muller PG. A comparison of repaglinide and glibenclamide in the treatment of type 2 diabetic patients previously treated with sulphonylureas. Eur J Clin Pharmacol 1999;55(3): 165–71.

[69] Marbury T, Huang WC, Strange P, Lebovitz H. Repaglinide versus glyburide: a one-year comparison trial. Diabetes Res Clin Pract 1999;43(3): 155–66.

[70] Moses R, Slobodniuk R, Boyages S, Colagiuri S, Kidson W, Carter J, et al. Effect of repaglinide addition to metformin monotherapy on glycemic control in patients with type 2 diabetes. Diabetes Care 1999;22(1):119–24.

[71] Raskin P, Jovanovic L, Berger S, Schwartz S, Woo V, Ratner R. Repaglinide/troglitazone combination therapy: improved glycemic control in type 2 diabetes. Diabetes Care 2000;23(7):979–83.

[72] Horton ES, Clinkingbeard C, Gatlin M, Foley J, Mallows S, Shen S. Nateglinide alone and in combination with metformin improves glycemic control by reducing mealtime glucose levels in type 2 diabetes. Diabetes Care 2000;23(11):1660–5.

[73] Bailey CJ, Turner RC. Metformin. N Engl J Med 1996;334(9):574–9.

[74] Kolata GB. The phenformin ban: is the drug an imminent hazard? Science 1979;203(4385):1094–6.

[75] Johansen K. Efficacy of metformin in the treatment of NIDDM. Meta-analysis. Diabetes Care 1999; 22(1):33–7.

[76] Stumvoll M, Nurjhan N, Perriello G, Dailey G, Gerich JE. Metabolic effects of metformin in non-insulin-dependent diabetes mellitus. N Engl J Med 1995;333(9):550–4.

[77] Kirpichnikov D, McFarlane SI, Sowers JR. Metformin: an update. Ann Intern Med 2002;137(1):25–33.

[78] Robinson AC, Burke J, Robinson S, Johnston DG, Elkeles RS. The effects of metformin on glycemic control and serum lipids in insulin-treated NIDDM patients with suboptimal metabolic control. Diabetes Care 1998;21(5):701–5.

[79] Murphy EJ, Davern TJ, Shakil AO, Shick L, Masharani U, Chow H, et al. Troglitazone-induced fulminant hepatic failure. Acute Liver Failure Study Group. Dig Dis Sci 2000;45(3):549–53.

[80] Scheen AJ, Lefebvre PJ. Troglitazone: antihyperglycemic activity and potential role in the treatment of type 2 diabetes. Diabetes Care 1999;22(9): 1568–77.

[81] Raskin P, Rappaport EB, Cole ST, Yan Y, Patwardhan R, Freed MI. Rosiglitazone short-term monotherapy lowers fasting and post-prandial glucose in patients with type II diabetes. Diabetologia 2000;43(3):278–84.

[82] Ghazzi MN, Perez JE, Antonucci TK, Driscoll JH, Huang SM, Faja BW, et al. Cardiac and glycemic benefits of troglitazone treatment in NIDDM. The Troglitazone Study Group. Diabetes 1997; 46(3):433–9.

[83] Nolan JJ, Ludvik B, Beerdsen P, Joyce M, Olefsky J. Improvement in glucose tolerance and insulin resistance in obese subjects treated with troglitazone. N Engl J Med 1994;331(18):1188–93.

[84] Prigeon RL, Kahn SE, Porte D Jr. Effect of troglitazone on B cell function, insulin sensitivity, and glycemic control in subjects with type 2 diabetes mellitus. J Clin Endocrinol Metab 1998;83(3): 819–23.

[85] Yamasaki Y, Kawamori R, Wasada T, Sato A, Omori Y, Eguchi H, et al. Pioglitazone (AD-4833) ameliorates insulin resistance in patients with NIDDM. AD-4833 Glucose Clamp Study Group, Japan. Tohoku J Exp Med 1997;183(3): 173–83.

[86] Bakst A, Schwartz S, Fischer JS. Avandia worldwide awareness registry: improved metabolic control with initiation of rosiglitazone in a diabetes clinic setting. Diabetes 2001;50(Suppl 2):A430. 6–26.

[87] Wagstaff AJ, Goa KL. Rosiglitazone: a review of its use in the management of type 2 diabetes mellitus. Drugs 2002;62(12):1805–37.

[88] Inzucchi SE, Maggs DG, Spollett GR, Page SL, Rife FS, Walton V, et al. Efficacy and metabolic effects of metformin and troglitazone in type II diabetes mellitus. N Engl J Med 1998;338(13): 867–72.

[89] Kersten S, Desvergne B, Wahli W. Roles of PPARs in health and disease. Nature 2000;405(6785): 421–4.

[90] Olefsky JM. Treatment of insulin resistance with peroxisome proliferator-activated receptor gamma agonists. J Clin Invest 2000;106(4):467–72.

[91] Mangelsdorf DJ, Thummel C, Beato M, Herrlich P, Schutz G, Umesono K, et al. The nuclear receptor superfamily: the second decade. Cell 1995; 83(6):835–9.

[92] Hu E, Tontonoz P, Spiegelman BM. Transdifferentiation of myoblasts by the adipogenic transcription factors PPAR gamma and C/EBP alpha. Proc Natl Acad Sci USA 1995;92(21):9856–60.

[93] Lemberger T, Braissant O, Juge-Aubry C, Keller H, Saladin R, Staels B, et al. PPAR tissue distribution and interactions with other hormone-signaling pathways. Ann N Y Acad Sci 1996;804:231–51.

[94] Kliewer SA, Forman BM, Blumberg B, Ong ES, Borgmeyer U, Mangelsdorf DJ, et al. Differential expression and activation of a family of murine peroxisome proliferator-activated receptors. Proc Natl Acad Sci USA 1994;91(15):7355–9.

[95] Ricote M, Huang J, Fajas L, Li A, Welch J, Najib J, et al. Expression of the peroxisome proliferator-activated receptor gamma (PPARgamma) in human atherosclerosis and regulation in macrophages by colony stimulating factors and oxidized low density lipoprotein. Proc Natl Acad Sci USA 1998;95(13): 7614–9.

[96] Marx N, Sukhova G, Murphy C, Libby P, Plutzky J. Macrophages in human atheroma contain PPARgamma: differentiation-dependent peroxisomal proliferator-activated receptor gamma(P-PARgamma) expression and reduction of MMP-9 activity through PPARgamma activation in mononuclear phagocytes in vitro. Am J Pathol 1998; 153(1):17–23.

[97] Viberti G, Kahn SE, Greene DA, Herman WH, Zinman B, Holman RR, et al. A diabetes outcome progression trial (ADOPT): an international multicenter study of the comparative efficacy of rosiglitazone, glyburide, and metformin in recently diagnosed type 2 diabetes. Diabetes Care 2002; 25(10):1737–43.

[98] Freed MI, Ratner R, Marcovina SM, Kreider MM, Biswas N, Cohen BR, et al. Effects of rosiglitazone alone and in combination with atorvastatin on the metabolic abnormalities in type 2 diabetes mellitus. Am J Cardiol 2002;90(9):947–52.

[99] Rosenblatt S, Miskin B, Glazer NB, Prince MJ, Robertson KE. The impact of pioglitazone on glycemic control and atherogenic dyslipidemia in patients with type 2 diabetes mellitus. Coron Artery Dis 2001;12(5):413–23.

[100] Suter SL, Nolan JJ, Wallace P, Gumbiner B, Olefsky JM. Metabolic effects of new oral hypoglycemic agent CS-045 in NIDDM subjects. Diabetes Care 1992;15(2):193–203.

[101] Troglitazone Study Group. The metabolic effects of troglitazone in non-insulin dependent diabetes (NIDDM) [abstract]. Diabetes 1997;46(Suppl 1): 149A.

[102] Prince MJ, Zagar AJ, Robertson KE. Effect of pioglitazone on HDL-C, a cardiovascular risk factor in type 2 diabetes [abstract]. Diabetes 2001; 50(Suppl 2):A128.

[103] Brown V. Detection and management of lipid disorders in diabetes. Diabetes Care 1996; (Suppl 1): S96–102.

[104] Ginsberg HN. Insulin resistance and cardiovascular disease. J Clin Invest 2000;106(4):453–8.

[105] Austin MA. Plasma triglyceride as a risk factor for coronary heart disease. The epidemiologic evidence and beyond. Am J Epidemiol 1989; 129(2):249–59.

[106] Chait A, Brazg RL, Tribble DL, Krauss RM. Susceptibility of small, dense, low-density lipoproteins to oxidative modification in subjects with the atherogenic lipoprotein phenotype, pattern B. Am J Med 1993;94(4):350–6.

[107] de Graaf J, Hak-Lemmers HL, Hectors MP, Demacker PN, Hendriks JC, Stalenhoef AF. Enhanced susceptibility to in vitro oxidation of the dense low density lipoprotein subfraction in

healthy subjects. Arterioscler Thromb 1991;11(2): 298–306.

[108] Lebovitz HE, Banerji MA. Insulin resistance and its treatment by thiazolidinediones. Recent Prog Horm Res 2001;56:265–94.

[109] Tack CJ, Smits P, Demacker PN, Stalenhoef AF. Troglitazone decreases the proportion of small, dense LDL and increases the resistance of LDL to oxidation in obese subjects. Diabetes Care 1998;21(5):796–9.

[110] Winkler K, Konrad T, Fullert S, Friedrich I, Destani R, Baumstark MW, et al. Pioglitazone reduces atherogenic dense LDL particles in nondiabetic patients with arterial hypertension: a double-blind, placebo-controlled study. Diabetes Care 2003;26(9):2588–94.

[111] Nagy L, Tontonoz P, Alvarez JG, Chen H, Evans RM. Oxidized LDL regulates macrophage gene expression through ligand activation of PPARgamma. Cell 1998;93(2):229–40.

[112] Chinetti G, Lestavel S, Bocher V, Remaley AT, Neve B, Torra IP, et al. PPAR-alpha and PPAR-gamma activators induce cholesterol removal from human macrophage foam cells through stimulation of the ABCA1 pathway. Nat Med 2001;7(1): 53–8.

[113] Tontonoz P, Nagy L, Alvarez JG, Thomazy VA, Evans RM. PPARgamma promotes monocyte/macrophage differentiation and uptake of oxidized LDL. Cell 1998;93(2):241–52.

[114] Raji A, Seely EW, Bekins SA, Williams GH, Simonson DC. Rosiglitazone improves insulin sensitivity and lowers blood pressure in hypertensive patients. Diabetes Care 2003;26(1):172–8.

[115] Ogihara T, Rakugi H, Ikegami H, Mikami H, Masuo K. Enhancement of insulin sensitivity by troglitazone lowers blood pressure in diabetic hypertensives. Am J Hypertens 1995;8(3):316–20.

[116] Bakris G, Viberti G, Weston WM, Heise M, Porter LE, Freed MI. Rosiglitazone reduces urinary albumin excretion in type II diabetes. J Hum Hypertens 2003;17(1):7–12.

[117] Scherbaun W, Göke B. For the German Pioglitazone Study Group. Pioglitazone reduces blood pressure in patients with type 2 diabetes mellitus diabetes. 2001;50:A462.

[118] Tack CJ, Ong MK, Lutterman JA, Smits P. Insulin-induced vasodilatation and endothelial function in obesity/insulin resistance. Effects of troglitazone. Diabetologia 1998;41(5):569–76.

[119] Song J, Walsh MF, Igwe R, Ram JL, Barazi M, Dominguez LJ, et al. Troglitazone reduces contraction by inhibition of vascular smooth muscle cell $Ca^{2+}$ currents and not endothelial nitric oxide production. Diabetes 1997;46(4):659–64.

[120] Morikang E, Benson SC, Kurtz TW, Pershadsingh HA. Effects of thiazolidinediones on growth and differentiation of human aorta and coronary myocytes. Am J Hypertens 1997;10(4 Pt 1):440–6.

[121] Zhang HY, Reddy SR, Kotchen TA. Antihypertensive effect of pioglitazone is not invariably associated with increased insulin sensitivity. Hypertension 1994;24(1):106–10.

[122] Buchanan TA, Meehan WP, Jeng YY, Yang D, Chan TM, Nadler JL, et al. Blood pressure lowering by pioglitazone. Evidence for a direct vascular effect. J Clin Invest 1995;96(1):354–60.

[123] Blackman DJ, Morris-Thurgood JA, Atherton JJ, Ellis GR, Anderson RA, Cockcroft JR, et al. Endothelium-derived nitric oxide contributes to the regulation of venous tone in humans. Circulation 2000;101(2):165–70.

[124] Tooke J. The association between insulin resistance and endotheliopathy. Diabetes Obes Metab 1999; 1(Suppl 1):S17–22.

[125] Vita JA, Frei B, Holbrook M, Gokce N, Leaf C, Keaney JF Jr. L-2-Oxothiazolidine-4-carboxylic acid reverses endothelial dysfunction in patients with coronary artery disease. J Clin Invest 1998; 101(6):1408–14.

[126] Dandona P, Aljada A, Mohanty P. The anti-inflammatory and potential anti-atherogenic effect of insulin: a new paradigm. Diabetologia 2002; 45(6):924–30.

[127] Avena R, Mitchell ME, Nylen ES, Curry KM, Sidawy AN. Insulin action enhancement normalizes brachial artery vasoactivity in patients with peripheral vascular disease and occult diabetes. J Vasc Surg 1998;28(6):1024–31.

[128] Mohanty P, Aljada A, Ghanim H, Tripathy D, Syed T, Hofmeyer D, et al. Rosiglitazone improves vascular reactivity, inhibits reactive oxygen species (ROS) generation, reduces p47$^{phox}$ subunit expression in mononuclear cells (MNC) and reduces C reactive protein (CRP) and monocyte chemotactic protein-1 (MCP1): evidence of a potent antiinflammatory effect [abstract]. Diabetes 2001;50(suppl 2): A68.

[129] Ohta MY, Nagai Y, Takamura T, Nohara E, Kobayashi K. Inhibitory effect of troglitazone on TNF-alpha-induced expression of monocyte chemoattractant protein-1 (MCP-1) in human endothelial cells. Diabetes Res Clin Pract 2000;48(3):171–6.

[130] Cominacini L, Garbin U, Pasini AF, Davoli A, Campagnola M, Rigoni A, et al. The expression of adhesion molecules on endothelial cells is inhibited by troglitazone through its antioxidant activity. Cell Adhes Commun 1999;7(3):223–31.

[131] Yoshimoto T, Naruse M, Shizume H, Naruse K, Tanabe A, Tanaka M, et al. Vasculo-protective effects of insulin sensitizing agent pioglitazone in neointimal thickening and hypertensive vascular hypertrophy. Atherosclerosis 1999;145(2):333–40.

[132] Kato K, Satoh H, Endo Y, Yamada D, Midorikawa S, Sato W, et al. Thiazolidinediones down-regulate plasminogen activator inhibitor type 1 expression in human vascular endothelial cells: a possible role for PPARgamma in endothelial

function. Biochem Biophys Res Commun 1999; 258(2):431–5.

[133] Ghanim H, Garg R, Aljada A, Mohanty P, Kumbkarni Y, Assian E, et al. Suppression of nuclear factor-kappaB and stimulation of inhibitor kappaB by troglitazone: evidence for an anti-inflammatory effect and a potential antiatherosclerotic effect in the obese. J Clin Endocrinol Metab 2001;86(3): 1306–12.

[134] Khandoudi N, Delerive P, Berrebi-Bertrand I, Buckingham RE, Staels B, Bril A. Rosiglitazone, a peroxisome proliferator-activated receptor-gamma, inhibits the Jun NH(2)-terminal kinase/activating protein 1 pathway and protects the heart from ischemia/reperfusion injury. Diabetes 2002;51(5):1507–14.

[135] Yue Tl TL, Chen J, Bao W, Narayanan PK, Bril A, Jiang W, et al. In vivo myocardial protection from ischemia/reperfusion injury by the peroxisome proliferator-activated receptor-gamma agonist rosiglitazone. Circulation 2001;104(21):2588–94.

[136] O'Leary DH, Polak JF, Kronmal RA, Manolio TA, Burke GL, Wolfson SK Jr. Carotid-artery intima and media thickness as a risk factor for myocardial infarction and stroke in older adults. Cardiovascular Health Study Collaborative Research Group. N Engl J Med 1999;340(1): 14–22.

[137] Minamikawa J, Tanaka S, Yamauchi M, Inoue D, Koshiyama H. Potent inhibitory effect of troglitazone on carotid arterial wall thickness in type 2 diabetes. J Clin Endocrinol Metab 1998;83(5): 1818–20.

[138] Koshiyama H, Shimono D, Kuwamura N, Minamikawa J, Nakamura Y. Rapid communication: inhibitory effect of pioglitazone on carotid arterial wall thickness in type 2 diabetes. J Clin Endocrinol Metab 2001;86(7):3452–6.

[139] Jiang C, Ting AT, Seed B. PPAR-gamma agonists inhibit production of monocyte inflammatory cytokines. Nature 1998;391(6662):82–6.

[140] Ehrmann DA, Schneider DJ, Sobel BE, Cavaghan MK, Imperial J, Rosenfield RL, et al. Troglitazone improves defects in insulin action, insulin secretion, ovarian steroidogenesis, and fibrinolysis in women with polycystic ovary syndrome. J Clin Endocrinol Metab 1997;82(7):2108–16.

[141] Fonseca VA, Diez J, McNamara DB. Decreasing restenosis following angioplasty: the potential of peroxisome proliferator-activated receptor gamma agonists. Diabetes Care 2004;27(11):2764–6.

[142] Weintraub WS, Stein B, Kosinski A, Douglas JS Jr, Ghazzal ZM, Jones EL, Morris DC, Guyton RA, Craver JM, King SB III. Outcome of coronary bypass surgery versus coronary angioplasty in diabetic patients with multivessel coronary artery disease. J Am Coll Cardiol 1998;31:10–9.

[143] Choi D, Kim SK, Choi SH. Preventative Effects of Rosiglitazone on Restenosis After Coronary Stent Implantation in Patients With Type 2 Diabetes. Diabetes Care 2004;27:2654–60.

[144] Takagi T, Yamamuro A, Tamita K, Yamabe K. Pioglitazone reduces neointimal tissue proliferation after coronary stent implantation in patients with type 2 diabetes mellitus: an intravascular ultrasound scanning study. Am Heart J 2003;146(2):E5.

[145] Davidson MB. Clinical implications of insulin resistance syndromes. Am J Med 1995;99(4):420–6.

[146] Nagi DK, Yudkin JS. Effects of metformin on insulin resistance, risk factors for cardiovascular disease, and plasminogen activator inhibitor in NIDDM subjects. A study of two ethnic groups. Diabetes Care 1993;16(4):621–9.

[147] Melidonis A, Stefanidis A, Tournis S, Manoussakis S, Handanis S, Zairis M, et al. The role of strict metabolic control by insulin infusion on fibrinolytic profile during an acute coronary event in diabetic patients. Clin Cardiol 2000;23(3):160–4.

[148] Sobel BE. Coronary artery disease and fibrinolysis: from the blood to the vessel wall. Thromb Haemost 1999;82(Suppl 1):8–13.

[149] Fonseca VA, Reynolds T, Hemphill D, Randolph C, Wall J, Valiquet TR, et al. Effect of troglitazone on fibrinolysis and activated coagulation in patients with non-insulin-dependent diabetes mellitus. J Diabetes Complications 1998;12(4):181–6.

[150] Kruszynska YT, Yu JG, Olefsky JM, Sobel BE. Effects of troglitazone on blood concentrations of plasminogen activator inhibitor 1 in patients with type 2 diabetes and in lean and obese normal subjects. Diabetes 2000;49(4):633–9.

[151] Nordt TK, Peter K, Bode C, Sobel BE. Differential regulation by troglitazone of plasminogen activator inhibitor type 1 in human hepatic and vascular cells. J Clin Endocrinol Metab 2000;85(4):1563–8.

[152] Freed M, Fuell D, Menci L, Heise M, Heise M. Effect of combination therapy with rosiglitazone and glibenclamide on PAI-1 antigen, PAI-1 activity, and tPA in patients with type 2 diabetes [abstract]. Diabetologia 2000;43(Suppl 1):A267.

[153] Ridker PM, Rifai N, Rose L, Buring JE, Cook NR. Comparison of C-reactive protein and low-density lipoprotein cholesterol levels in the prediction of first cardiovascular events. N Engl J Med 2002; 347(20):1557–65.

[154] Fuell DL, Freed MI, Greenberg AS, Haffner S, Chen H. The effect of treatment with rosiglitazone on C-reactive protein and interleukin-6 in patients with Type 2 diabetes [abstract]. Diabetes 2001; 50(Suppl 2):A435.

[155] Haffner SM, Greenberg AS, Weston WM, Chen H, Williams K, Freed MI. Effect of rosiglitazone treatment on nontraditional markers of cardiovascular disease in patients with type 2 diabetes mellitus. Circulation 2002;106(6):679–84.

[156] Mohanty P, Aljada A, Ghanim H, et al. Evidence for a potent antiinflammatory effect of rosiglitazone. J Clin Endocrinol Metab 2004;89(6):2728–35.

[157] Imano E, Kanda T, Nakatani Y, Nishida T, Arai K, Motomura M, et al. Effect of troglitazone on micro-albuminuria in patients with incipient diabetic nephropathy. Diabetes Care 1998;21(12):2135–9.

[158] Mattock MB, Morrish NJ, Viberti G, Keen H, Fitzgerald AP, Jackson G. Prospective study of microalbuminuria as predictor of mortality in NIDDM. Diabetes 1992;41(6):736–41.

[159] Lebovitz HE, Dole JF, Patwardhan R, Rappaport EB, Freed MI. Rosiglitazone monotherapy is effective in patients with type 2 diabetes. J Clin Endocrinol Metab 2001;86(1):280–8.

[160] Nicholas SB, Kawano Y, Wakino S, Collins AR, Hsueh WA. Expression and function of peroxisome proliferator-activated receptor-gamma in mesangial cells. Hypertension 2001;37(2 Part 2):722–7.

[161] Fonseca V, Foyt HL, Shen K, Whitcomb R. Long-term effects of troglitazone: open-label extension studies in type 2 diabetic patients. Diabetes Care 2000;23(3):354–9.

[162] Mori Y, Murakawa Y, Okada K, Horikoshi H, Yokoyama J, Tajima N, et al. Effect of troglitazone on body fat distribution in type 2 diabetic patients. Diabetes Care 1999;22(6):908–12.

[163] Patel J, Anderson RJ, Rappaport EB. Rosiglitazone monotherapy improves glycaemic control in patients with type 2 diabetes: a twelve-week, randomized, placebo-controlled study. Diabetes Obes Metab 1999;1(3):165–72.

[164] Spiegelman BM. PPAR-gamma: adipogenic regulator and thiazolidinedione receptor. Diabetes 1998;47(4):507–14.

[165] Akazawa S, Sun F, Ito M, Kawasaki E, Eguchi K. Efficacy of troglitazone on body fat distribution in type 2 diabetes. Diabetes Care 2000;23(8):1067–71.

[166] Kelly IE, Han TS, Walsh K, Lean ME. Effects of a thiazolidinedione compound on body fat and fat distribution of patients with type 2 diabetes. Diabetes Care 1999;22(2):288–93.

[167] Nakamura T, Funahashi T, Yamashita S, Nishida M, Nishida Y, Takahashi M, et al. Thiazolidinedione derivative improves fat distribution and multiple risk factors in subjects with visceral fat accumulation—double-blind   placebo-controlled trial. Diabetes Res Clin Pract 2001;54(3):181–90.

[168] Carey DG, Jenkins AB, Campbell LV, Freund J, Chisholm DJ. Abdominal fat and insulin resistance in normal and overweight women: Direct measurements reveal a strong relationship in subjects at both low and high risk of NIDDM. Diabetes 1996;45(5):633–8.

[169] Kissebah AH, Krakower GR. Regional adiposity and morbidity. Physiol Rev 1994;74(4): 761–811.

[170] Carey DG, Cowin GJ, Galloway GJ, Jones NP, Richards JC, Biswas N, et al. Effect of rosiglitazone on insulin sensitivity and body composition in type 2 diabetic patients. Obes Res 2002;10(10):1008–15.

[171] Miyazaki Y, Mahankali A, Matsuda M, Mahankali S, Hardies J, Cusi K, et al. Effect of pioglitazone on abdominal fat distribution and insulin sensitivity in type 2 diabetic patients. J Clin Endocrinol Metab 2002;87(6):2784–91.

[172] The Bypass Angioplasty Revascularization Investigation (BARI) Investigators. Protocol for the Bypass Angioplasty Revascularization Investigation. Circulation 1991;84(Suppl V):V1–27.

[173] Comparison of coronary bypass surgery with angioplasty in patients with multivessel disease. The Bypass Angioplasty Revascularization Investigation (BARI) Investigators. N Engl J Med 1996; 335(4):217–25.

[174] Seven-year outcome in the Bypass Angioplasty Revascularization Investigation (BARI) by treatment and diabetic status. J Am Coll Cardiol 2000;35(5): 1122–9.

[175] BARI2D trial. Available at http://www.bari2D. org.

[176] Erle G, Lovise S, Stocchiero C, Lora L, Coppini A, Marchetti P, et al. A comparison of preconstituted, fixed combinations of low-dose glyburide plus metformin versus high-dose glyburide alone in the treatment of type 2 diabetic patients. Acta Diabetol 1999;36(1–2):61–5.

[177] DeFronzo RA, Goodman AM. Efficacy of metformin in patients with non-insulin-dependent diabetes mellitus. The Multicenter Metformin Study Group. N Engl J Med 1995;333(9):541–9.

[178] Horton ES, Whitehouse F, Ghazzi MN, Venable TC, Whitcomb RW. Troglitazone in combination with sulfonylurea restores glycemic control in patients with type 2 diabetes. The Troglitazone Study Group. Diabetes Care 1998;21(9):1462–9.

[179] Wolffenbuttel BH, Gomis R, Squatrito S, Jones NP, Patwardhan RN. Addition of low-dose rosiglitazone to sulphonylurea therapy improves glycaemic control in Type 2 diabetic patients. Diabet Med 2000;17(1):40–7.

ELSEVIER
SAUNDERS

Cardiol Clin 23 (2005) 139–152

CARDIOLOGY
CLINICS

# Diabetes and Hypertension, the Deadly Duet: Importance, Therapeutic Strategy, and Selection of Drug Therapy

## Prakash C. Deedwania, MD, FACC, FACP, FCCP, FAHA*

*Department of Medicine, VA Central California Health Care System/University Medical Center, University of California, San Francisco Program at Fresno, 2615 East Clinton Avenue (111), Fresno, CA 93703, USA*

Diabetes and hypertension often coexist and are two of the most common clinical conditions that are encountered in clinical practice. Both of these conditions significantly increase the risk of cardiovascular (CV) morbidity and mortality [1,2]. Several recent studies showed that appropriate treatment of patients who have diabetes and hypertension can significantly reduce the risk of CV events and improve long-term outcome [3–5]. Prevalence of diabetes is greater than 7% to 8% in adults in the United States [6]. Recent trends show a steady increase in prevalence, especially in non-Caucasian ethnic groups, and it is likely to continue to increase with the increasing number of elderly and obese individuals in the United States population. Diabetes consumes about 12% of total health care costs ($100 billion per year). The prevalence of hypertension in type 2 diabetic patients is about two times that observed in general populations [7–9]. The prevalence of hypertension (blood pressure [BP] ≥ 160/ 90 mm Hg) was approximately 39% in type 2 diabetic patients who were between age 25 and 64 in the United Kingdom Prospective Diabetes Study Group (UKPDS) [8].

Coexistence of diabetes and hypertension increases the risk of coronary artery disease (CAD) mortality by more than threefold and twofold in younger and older diabetic patients, respectively [10]. Hypertension and diabetes act synergistically in the development of CV complications [11–12]. Most diabetics (up to 80%) die of CV

complications [1]. Hypertension in diabetic patients contributes to diabetic nephropathy and retinopathy and increases the risk of macrovascular complications, such as myocardial infarction, congestive heart failure, and stroke [3]. Hypertension may contribute to up to 75% of diabetes-related CV complications [13]. Treatment of hypertension resulted in a 76% reduction in CV mortality in elderly diabetic patients who had systolic hypertension [14]. Furthermore, diabetes mellitus and hypertension account for the vast majority of end-stage renal disease (ESRD). After ESRD develops in patients who have diabetes, the 5-year survival rates are 5% in Germany and 27% in Australia [15].

The data from several recent studies indicate that BP control is more effective in reducing diabetic macrovascular complications than glycemic control [3–5,16]. The analysis of the UKPDS [17] data showed that tight control of BP in diabetic patients who had hypertension is highly effective in reducing CV complications and is a cost-effective therapeutic strategy. Simulation model analysis demonstrated that aggressive BP control (<130/85 mm Hg) was cost effective in diabetic patients who had hypertension [18]. These findings are not surprising because hypertension has a significantly greater impact on CV morbidity and mortality in diabetic patients than in nondiabetic patients. The data from National Health and Nutrition Examination Survey in the United States III (1991–1994) showed that only 53% of hypertensive patients received treatment; only 27% of them had BP that was less than 140/ 90 mm Hg [19]. A more recent population-based

---

* Corresponding author.
*E-mail address:* deed@ucsfresno.edu

0733-8651/05/$ - see front matter © 2005 Elsevier Inc. All rights reserved.
doi:10.1016/j.ccl.2004.06.006

study from Italy showed that among hypertensive elderly patients, 60% were being treated; however, only 10.5% had their hypertension controlled with BP that was less than 140/90 mm Hg [20]. It is well-known that hypertension is more difficult to control in diabetic patients [21] and often requires multiple antihypertensive drugs [3]. To achieve a BP that is less than 130/80 mm Hg in diabetics, as recommended by the Joint National Committee (JNC) VII, American Diabetes Association (ADA) [22], and Canadian Medical Association (CMA) [23], vigorous efforts should be made by the clinicians that often requires initiation of treatment with a combination therapy and titrating the drugs to their maximum dosage.

The availability of newer drugs, as well as the data from several large, randomized controlled clinical trials (RCTs), have made significant contributions to the selection of the most appropriate therapy for management of patients who have diabetes and hypertension. Although drugs, such as α-adrenergic antagonists (AAAs) and calcium-channel blockers (CCBs), were recommended in the past, they are not considered suitable as first-line therapy today. The JNC VII guidelines [19] recommend the target BP to be less than 130/85 mm Hg in diabetics who have hypertension. Based on the data from recent studies, the ADA [33] and CMA [23] have pushed the target BP to be even lower, with diastolic BP of less than 80. The following section provides an overview of the clinical trials that support these recommendations as well as a definition of the role of various drugs in the treatment of hypertension in the setting of diabetes.

**Individual drug review**

*Angiotensin-converting enzyme inhibitors*

Angiotensin-converting-enzyme (ACE) inhibitors are the initial drug choice for patients who have diabetes and hypertension, especially those who have albuminuria. Although initially recommended based on a small set of data, several recent RCTs clearly support the use of ACE inhibitors based on their favorable impact on CV and renal outcomes.

ACE is responsible for the conversion of angiotensin I to angiotensin II, which elevates BP by direct vasoconstriction as well as salt and water retention due to increased aldosterone secretion. ACE inhibitors block production of angiotensin II and degradation of bradykinin, and as a result, decrease the BP [24,25]. ACE

inhibitors also reduce insulin resistance. ACE inhibitors decreased the incidence of new-onset diabetes mellitus in the Captopril Prevention Project (CAPPP) [26] and the Heart Outcomes Prevention Evaluation (HOPE) [27] studies. This is believed to occur secondary to improved insulin sensitivity, which also might result in better glycemic control in diabetic patients [28,29]. No large, randomized, placebo-controlled trial involved only diabetic patients with ACE inhibitors. Nevertheless, the benefit of ACE inhibitors in diabetic patients who had hypertension was well-illustrated in the HOPE trial. In the HOPE [27,30] study, 56% of the subjects were hypertensive and 39% were diabetic. The HOPE study demonstrated that the benefits of ACE inhibitors extend far beyond BP reduction. Although the reduction in mean BP was only 2.4/1.0 mm Hg with ramipril during the 4.5-year study period, there was an impressive 37% risk reduction in death from CV causes and a 24% decrease in all-cause mortality [30]. There also was a 16% decrease in the combined risk of overt nephropathy, dialysis, and laser therapy. These data suggest that ACE inhibitors have additional vasculoprotective and cardioprotective effects. Whether the cardioprotective effect is mediated, in part, by reducing insulin resistance is not clear.

Generally, ACE inhibitors are well-tolerated; hyperkalemia (mostly in patients who have renal insufficiency) [31], renal failure (in patients who have bilateral renal artery stenosis), and angioedema were the most severe, but rarely-reported, adverse effects for the entire class (Table 1). The bradykinin-potentiating effect of ACE inhibitors [32] is responsible for the annoying cough that is secondary to ACE inhibitors and that occurs in up to 10% of patients [33]. There is no evidence that one ACE inhibitor is better than the others, but it is reasonable to choose the one that has the longer half-life and lower cost. Trandolapril, fosinopril, ramipril, and enalapril have average trough-peak ratios of 50% or greater [34], which may give a better BP control between dosing intervals. Because of the recent uniform pricing structure for some ACE inhibitors (regardless of the dose strengths), they may be less expensive when a higher dose is required or when the tablet is scored (Table 2). Generic captopril and enalapril also have become available with some cost advantage (see Table 2). Captopril has the disadvantages of multiple daily dosing and the rare adverse effects, such as neutropenia, nephrotic syndrome, and rashes, from its unique sulfhydryl group [37].

**Table 1**
The major differences in side effects between angiotensin-converting enzyme inhibitors and angiotensin II–receptor blockers

| | ACE-I | ARBs | Investigators |
|---|---|---|---|
| Bradykinin | Increased | No change | Goodfriend et al, 1996 [32] |
| Cough | 10% | No | Wright, 2000 [33] |
| Angioedema | 0.1–0.5% | <0.1–0.5% | Warner et al, 2000 [35]; grossman, 2000 [36] |
| Hyperkalemia in patients who have renal failure | Common | May be less common | Bakris et al, 2000 [37] |

*Abbreviations:* ACE-I, angiotensin-converting enzyme inhibitor; ARBS, angiotensin II–receptor blockers.

## Thiazide diuretics

Thiazide diuretics (TDs) increase the sodium chloride secretion in renal distal tubules. Their antihypertensive effects are not fully understood, but it is believed that TDs decrease BP by reducing plasma volume and peripheral resistance [38]. It is known that hypertensive, diabetic patients are salt sensitive and have increased peripheral vascular resistance [39]. Theoretically, TDs should work well in this group of patients because of their vasodilatory and diuretic effects. In the Systolic Hypertension in the Elderly Program (SHEP) trial, the CV event rate was reduced by 34% in hypertensive, diabetic patients who were assigned randomly to low-dosage

chlorthalidone [40]. Diabetic patients benefited twice as much as nondiabetic patients from low-dosage chlorthalidone. The magnitudes of benefit may be underestimated because some patients who were assigned to the placebo group also received active therapy. Further analysis indicated that benefits in the treatment group were not attributable to the step 2 drugs (atenolol or to reserpine) in the overall group of hypertensives [41]. Subgroup analysis to evaluate the impact of atenolol in diabetics was not possible because of the small sample size. The major adverse effects from high-dosage TDs are hypokalemia, hyperglycemia, and increased cholesterol. These effects are much less a concern when a low dosage is used [40]. An early observational study showed

**Table 2**
Price comparison of selected combination drugs for hypertension

| Agent 1 | Price of 30 tablets ($) | Agent 2 | Price of 30 tablets ($) | Name of combination pill | Price of combination pill 30 tablets ($) |
|---|---|---|---|---|---|
| Chlorthalidone, 25 mg | 5.62 | Atenolol, 50 mg[a] | 4.29 | Atenolol-Chlorthalidone[a] | 11.41 |
| HCTZ, 12.5 mg capsule | 13.08 | Valsartan, 80 mg[a] | 38.80 | Diovan HCT[a] | 41.03 |
| HCTZ, 12.5 mg capsule | 13.08 | Irbesartan, 150 mg | 39.87 | Avalide[a] | 45.83 |
| HCTZ, 12.5 mg capsule | 13.08 | Losartan, 50 mg | 36.39 | Hyzaar | 38.23 |
| HCTZ, 25 mg tablet | 4.98[b] | Benazepril, 20 mg[a] | 23.13 | Lotensin HCT[a] | 24.30 |
| HCTZ, 12.5 mg capsule | 13.08 | Zestril, 10 mg | 51.23[c] | Zestoretic | 31.47 |
| HCTZ, 12.5 mg capsule | 13.08 | Enalapril, 10 mg | 9.54 | Vaseretic | 38.80 |
| Felodipine, 5 mg | 31.77 | Enalapril, 5 mg | 24.10[c] | Lexxel[a] | 41.01 |
| Amlodipine, 5 mg | 35.02 | Benezepril, 10 mg | 23.13 | Lotrel | 51.14 |
| Verapamil | 7.98 | Trandolapril, 2 mg[a] | 25.76 | Tarka[a] | 51.20 |
| | | Fosinopril, 20 mg[a] | 50.32[c] | | |
| | | Ramipril, 5 mg | 53.92 | | |
| | | Captopril, 50 mg | 7.64[c] | | |

*Abbreviation:* HCTZ, hydrochlorothiazide.
[a] Very close or same price for different dosages.
[b] HCTZ, 25 mg, tablet can be split; 90 tablets of 25 mg or 50 mg cost $5.49.
[c] The price is for 60 tablets.
*Data from* www.drugstore.com/pharmacy/prices.

increased mortality in diabetic patients who received high-dosage TDs [42]. The most likely explanation was increased risk of fatal arrhythmia due to hypokalemia that was secondary to TDs [43].

### β-Blockers

β-Blockers (βBs) have been used in the treatment of hypertension for a long time. Although based on some studies, JNC V and VI recommended βBs as first-line therapy for hypertension; however, a recent meta-analysis raised some question by showing a marginal, but statistically insignificant, effect of βBs on CV morbidity and mortality in hypertensive patients [25]. βB–placebo-controlled trials are not available in diabetic patients who have hypertension; however, because most diabetic patients die of CV complications, βBs should be considered strongly in hypertensive, diabetic patients. Atenolol was as effective as ACE inhibitors in reducing CV morbidity and mortality in diabetic, hypertensive patients in the UKPDS [3,5]. βBs also are preferable in diabetic patients who have CAD and always should be used in the postinfarction period because compared with nondiabetic patients, there is a significantly greater cardioprotective effect of βBs in diabetics [44]. Additionally, based on recent data, diabetic patients who have heart failure should be given βB therapy in addition to ACE inhibitor therapy.

A few unfavorable metabolic effects of βBs were reported. βBs might exacerbate glucose intolerance [5,45,46], increase triglycerides, and decrease high-density lipoproteins [47]. These effects on surrogate end points should not prevent us from using βBs in diabetic patients who have hypertension. Caution should be taken when using βBs in diabetic patients who are at risk for severe hypoglycemia, although there is no convincing evidence that β1-selective blockers increase the risk of masking hypoglycemia symptoms [48–50]. High dosages of selective β1-blockers should be avoided in patients who have asthma or severe obstructive lung diseases. βBs should not be used in patients who have advanced heart block or sinus node disease without a pacemaker.

### Calcium-channel blockers

CCBs have a neutral effect on carbohydrate metabolism [51] and low side-effect profiles. Subgroup analysis of elderly diabetic patients who had systolic hypertension from a placebo-controlled trial (systolic hypertension in Europe trial investigators) clearly showed an impressive CV morbidity and total mortality reduction in the group that received nitrendipine alone [14]. Another large study, the Hypertension Optimal Treatment (HOT), demonstrated that the intensive control of BP, reduced the CV events more significantly than in the group whose BP was less tightly controlled [52]. The beneficial effects were of significantly greater magnitude in the diabetic cohort; however, many of the diabetic patients also received ACE inhibitors. Other recent studies, however, such as the Fosinopril/Amlodipine Event Trial (FACET) [53] and the Appropriate Blood Pressure Control in Diabetes (ABCD) [54] trials, showed that compared with ACE inhibitors, treatment with dihydropyridine CCBs in diabetic hypertensive patients might be harmful. This raised significant concern about the safety of dihydropyridine CCBs in these patients. Overall, CCBs are well-tolerated; the major side effects are headache, flushing, and ankle edema [55].

### α-Adrenergic antagonists

AAAs decrease insulin resistance and cholesterol [56,57]. Theoretically, this class of drug may improve glycemic control in patients who have diabetes and improve long-term outcome. Findings from the Antihypertensive and Lipid Lowering Treatment to Prevent Heart Attack Trial (ALLHAT), however, showed that patients who were on doxazosin had a higher risk of developing congestive heart failure, angina, and stroke than patients who were assigned to chlorthalidone [58]. The most plausible explanation is that these adverse effects occurred because AAAs increase plasma volume [59] and norepinephrine [60]. In addition, AAAs are less likely to regress left ventricular mass [61,62]. Based on the results of the ALLHAT, doxazosin should not be used as first-line drug for hypertension. Furthermore, it is recommended that βBs, in combination with a diuretic, should be added to α-adrenergic blockers in hypertensive, diabetic patients who are being treated for benign prostate hypertrophy. Alternatively, prostate-selective α-adrenergic blockers may be considered.

### Angiotensin II–receptor blockers

It is well-known that the production of angiotensin II may not be blocked completely by ACE inhibitors because of the formation of angiotensin II by the non-ACE–dependent pathway [63]. Angiotensin II–receptor blockers (ARBs) act by blocking the effects of angiotensin II on angiotensin I receptors, and therefore, provide more complete blockade to the action of angiotensin II, regardless of its origin. Recently, the combination of ACE inhibitors and ARBs was more effective in decreasing BP and reducing proteinuria than either agent alone [64]. Another study showed that as monotherapy, ACE inhibitors and ARBs decreased the BP and urine protein to the same extent in diabetic patients who had hypertension [65]. In general, ARBs have a better side-effect profile than ACE inhibitors (see Table 1). In a recent trial, irbesartan was superior to amlodipine in improving creatinine clearance and reducing proteinuria in diabetic patients who had hypertension, despite similar antihypertensive effects [66].

### Selection of antihypertensive drug in diabetes mellitus

ACE inhibitors, nondihydropyridine CCBs, TDs, and βBs reduced CV complications in patients who had diabetes and hypertension in several long-term, large, RCTs (Tables 3 and 4). Limited data is available with direct comparisons of various drugs in diabetic, hypertensive patients (Table 5).

There was no convincing evidence from several large RCTs (eg, CAPPP [26], Swedish Trial in Old Patients with Hypertension 2 [STOP-2] [68], Nordic Diltiazem [NORDIL] study [69], and Intervention as a Goal in Hypertension Treatment [INSIGHT] [70]) that newer agents, such as ACE inhibitors and CCBs, are better than diuretics and βBs in reducing CV events in treating hypertension in the general population. Because diabetes is an important and independent risk factor for CV morbidity and mortality and because most diabetics die of CV complications [1], subgroup analysis of diabetic, hypertensive patients in these trials revealed that most required multiple drugs for adequate control of their BP.

### Angiotensin-converting enzyme inhibitors versus other agents

In the CAPPP trial, diabetic patients who were on captopril had less cardiac mortality and all-cause mortality than did those who were on βBs or TDs [26]. The report did not further divide the impact of captopril over βBs or TDs. However, the STOP-2 did not find any difference in major CV events and total mortality among patients who were randomized to TDs/βBs versus ACE inhibitors versus CCBs [67], although there was a statistically significant reduction in myocardial infarction (MI) in those who were on ACE inhibitors compared with those who received CCBs (see Table 5). The data from CAPPP and STOP-2 are based on post hoc analysis because only a small percentage of participants were diabetic; thus, such analyses may suffer from inherited bias (eg, violation of randomization). In contrast, the UKPDS, ABCD, and FACET trials included only diabetic patients who had hypertension. Results from these three trials seem to be more convincing in favor of ACE inhibitor use in diabetic patients. The UKPDS demonstrated

Table 3

Subgroup analysis of effects of antihypertensive agents on cardiovascular complications in type 2 diabetes in randomized, placebo-controlled trials

| Trial | N (% of patients who had DM-2) | Agents | Duration (y) | CV events[a] RR | MI RR | Stroke RR | Total mortality RR |
|---|---|---|---|---|---|---|---|
| SHEP [40] | 4736 (12.3) | Chlorthalidone Atenolol[b] | 5 | 0.66[a] | 0.46[c] | 0.78 | 0.74 |
| SYST-EUR [14] | 4695 (10.5) | Nitrendipine | 2 | 0.31[c] | 0.37[c,d] | 0.27[c] | 0.45[c] |
| HOPE [30] | 9297 (38.5) | Ramipril | 4.5 | 0.77[c] | 0.9[c] | 0.69[c] | 0.77[c] |

Relative risks of outcomes for active treatment compared with placebo.

*Abbreviations:* DM-2, diabetes mellitus type 2; MI, myocardial infarction; RR, relative risk; SYST-EUR, Systolic Hypertension in Europe Trial.

[a] CV events include myocardial infarction, sudden cardiac death, revascularization, and stroke.

[b] Atenolol was added if chlorthalidone was not effective.

[c] Statistically significant.

[d] For cardiac events.

Table 4

The effect of tight versus less tight blood pressure control on cardiovascular complications in type 2 diabetes in randomized, active-controlled trials

| Trial | N (% who had DM) | Agents | Baseline BP (mm Hg) | Achieved BP (mm Hg) | Duration (y) | CV events | MI | Stroke | Total death |
|---|---|---|---|---|---|---|---|---|---|
| UKPDS [3] | 1148 (100) | Captopril or atenolol | T 159/94 LT 160/94 | 144/82 154/87 | 9 | ↓↓ | ↓ | ↓↓ | ↓ |
| ABCD [67][a] | 470 (100) | Nisoldipine or enalapril | T 156/98 LT 154/98 | 132/78 138/86 | 5.3 | NE | NE | NE | ↓↓ |
| HOT [52] | 18,790 (8.0) | Felodipine | 170/105 | 140/81 | 3.8 | ↓↓ | ↓ | ↓ | ↓ |

*Abbreviations:* ↓, statistically nonsignificant reduction; ↓↓, statistically significant reduction; LT, less tight; NE, no effect; T, tight.

[a] Patients were assigned randomly to tight or less tight control groups. Within each group, patients were treated further randomly with nisoldipine or enalapril. The comparison in this table was between moderate and intensive therapy instead of between nisoldipine and enalapril as shown in Table 3.

that the benefit that was achieved with captopril was similar to that of atenolol; however, captopril was only given once or twice daily; this may account partially for its lack of superiority over atenolol. Thirty-six percent of patients who received atenolol and 27% patients who received captopril also received nifedipine to achieve target BP control in the UKPDS [5]. This also might make it difficult to determine the difference between various treatments. ACE inhibitors were superior to dihydropyridine CCBs in randomized head-to-head comparator studies, such as the ABCD and the FACET trials (see Table 5) [53,54]. Thirty-one percent of patients who received fosinopril received additional amlodipine, whereas fosinopril was added to 26% of patients who received amlodipine in the FACET trial. This may underestimate the benefits of fosinopril. The results of these two trials also raised significant concern regarding the safety of dihydropyridine CCBs in diabetic, hypertensive patients. Generally, it is not recommended that dihydropyridine CCBs be used as initial therapy in diabetic, hypertensive subjects.

Table 5

Head-to-head comparison of antihypertensive agents in randomized, actively-controlled trials in type 2 diabetic patients who had hypertension

| Trial | N (# who had DM) | Agents | Years | CV events | MI (95% Confidence Interval) | Stroke | Total mortality |
|---|---|---|---|---|---|---|---|
| UKPDS [3] | 1148 (1148) | Captopril vs atenolol | 9 | Not reported | 1.2 (0.82–1.76) | 1.12 (0.59–2.12) | 1.14 (0.81–1.61) |
| ABCD [53] | 470 (470) | Enalapril vs nisoldipine | 5 | 0.43 (0.25–0.73) | 0.18 (0.07–0.48) | 0.63 (0.24–1.67) | 0.77 (0.36–1.67) |
| FACET [54] | 380 (380) | Fosinopril vs amlodipine | 2.8 | 0.49 (0.26–0.95) | 0.77 (0.34–1.75) | 0.39 (0.12–1.23) | 0.81 (0.22–3.02) |
| CAPPP [26] | 10985 (572) | Captopril vs diuretics, βB | 6.1 | 0.59 (0.38–0.91) | 0.34 (0.17–0.67) | 1.02 (0.55–1.88) | 0.54 (0.31–0.96) |
| STOP-2 [67] | 6614 (466) | ACE-Is vs CCBs[a] | 4 | 0.94 (0.67–1.32) | 0.51 (0.28–0.92) | 1.16 (0.71–1.91) | 1.14 (0.78–1.67) |
| STOP-2 [67] | 6614 (488) | ACE-Is vs diuretics or βB[a] | 4 | 0.85 (0.62–1.18) | 0.68 (0.37–1.26) | 0.88 (0.56–1.40) | 0.88 (0.62–1.26) |

Relative risks compared ACE inhibitors with other agents.

[a] In the STOP-2 trial, βBs included atenolol, metoprolol, and pindolol; CCBs were felopipine and isradipine; and ACE inhibitors included enalapril and lisinopril.

*Calcium-channel blockers versus other agents*

Trials that have compared CCBs, diuretics, and βBs are limited. Diltiazem was compared with diuretics and βBs in the NORDIL trial that involved 10,881 hypertensive patients. There was a slight, but statistically significant, decreased incidence of stroke in the group that received diltiazem, despite the fact that the achieved systolic BP was 3 mm Hg higher in that group. Although the study was not designed to compare these three classes of agents independently, the post hoc analysis of 727 participants who had diabetes mellitus did not show any difference in CV-related outcomes between the diltiazem-based therapeutic regimen and a TD or βB regimen [69]. Conversely, more fatal MIs and heart failure were noted in patients who received nifedipine compared with diuretics in the INSIGHT trial [70]. Nevertheless, the total mortality was the same and the subgroup analysis of diabetic patients was not reported. Moreover, the high drop-out rate in the INSIGHT study makes the results difficult to interpret. Furthermore, the STOP-2 trial did not find any difference in major CV events and total mortality among diabetic patients who were randomized to TDs/βBs versus CCB in a post hoc analysis [67]. In summary, although these three trials do not provide an unequivocal answer regarding the selection of the best agent among CCBs, TDs, and βBs in diabetic patients, based on the results of the FACET and the ABCD trials it is well-accepted that dihydropyridine CCBs should not be used as first-line therapy in diabetic, hypertensive patients.

*Surrogate markers*

Selection of an antihypertensive agent should be based on the effects of the given agent on hard outcomes, such as CV mortality and total mortality, rather than on its metabolic or surrogate effects. For example, despite the unfavorable metabolic effects of TDs or βBs, these drugs are preferred over AAAs based on their long-term morbidity and mortality benefits. The available data (see Table 5) suggest that ACE inhibitors should be the agents of choice in diabetics who have hypertension. Although it usually is considered that βBs should be the first choice in hypertensive diabetics who have CAD, the recent data from the HOPE study suggests that an ACE inhibitor also should be used to achieve maximum

cardioprotection. TDs and CCBs can be the add-on agents if the BP is still uncontrolled.

*Agents of choice in diabetic patients who have renal failure*

ACE inhibitors and ARBs are the only drugs that have been proven to reduce the ESRD and death in diabetic patients who have renal failure. In the landmark study by Lewis et al [71], captopril was able to reduce the rate of end-stage renal failure and death in patients who had type 1 diabetes and hypertension by 50%. The role of ACE inhibitors in patients who have type 2 diabetes and renal failure is not-well defined; only a few, small-scale studies have evaluated their role. Treatment with enalapril slowed down the increase in serum creatinine and stopped the increase in urine albumin excretion in normo-albuminuric [72] and microalbuminuric [73] diabetic patients who did not have hypertension. Because of the small sample size and short-term follow-up period, these studies were unable to evaluate the effectiveness of ACE inhibitors on the development of end-stage renal failure. Also, because the control groups only received placebo, it is not clear if the benefit was due to a BP decreasing effect or the specific effect of ACE inhibitors on kidney function [74]. The data from evaluation of surrogates, such as proteinuria, are, however, convincing. For example, in the SHEP trial, TD therapy slowed the development of proteinuria in diabetic, hypertensive patients [40]. More recently, in the HOPE study [27,30], ramipril had antiproteinuric effect. Comparative data regarding the benefits of various antihypertensive drugs are lacking. More recent data in the UKPDS did not substantiate the superiority of captopril over atenolol in regards to proteinuria and renal protection in patients who had type 2 diabetes [3,5].

In contrast, several large-scale RCTs demonstrated the benefit of ARBs in patients who had early- or late-stage diabetic nephropathy and type 2 diabetes [74]. Based on these results, it has been recommended that ARBs, as a class, should be the therapy of choice for most diabetic patients who have microalbuminuria or advanced nephropathy. No head-to-head comparison has been made in any RCT between ACE inhibitors and ARBs in diabetic patients who have nephropathy. Such studies are needed; some investigators believe that ACE inhibitors are overall superior agents for diabetic patients because of their vasculoprotective effects.

ACE inhibitors also were superior to dihydropyridine CCBs on CV end points in diabetic patients who did not have kidney failure [53,54]. Based on these facts, it seems reasonable to consider ACE inhibitors as the first-line drug for diabetic, hypertensive patients who have albuminuria.

## What is the optimal target blood pressure?

JNC VII [19] recommends the target BP to be less than 130/85 mm Hg in diabetics who have hypertension. The ADA [22] and the CMA [23] have pushed the target even lower, with a goal for diastolic BP of less than 80 mm Hg. What is the evidence for these recommendations? Three, randomized, actively-controlled trials provided some direct evidence regarding the need for aggressive BP control (see Table 4) [3,52,75].

The intensive BP control in UKPDS 38 [3] trial was achieved at a target of 144/82 mm Hg. Compared with conventional control (BP 154/87 mm Hg), there was a 32%, 44%, and 37% reduction of diabetes-related death, stroke, and microvascular complications, respectively. For a 10 mm Hg greater reduction in systolic BP, there was a significantly greater reduction in the risk of CV end points, including MI and heart failure.

In the ABCD trial [75], 470 patients who had type 2 diabetes with a baseline BP of approximately 155/98 mm Hg were assigned randomly to intensive BP control (achieved 132/78 mm Hg) or less tight control (achieved 138/86 mm Hg). There was a 49% reduction in the intensive BP control group in all-cause mortality; however, this benefit was not due to differences in MI, cerebrovascular events, or congestive heart failure. The J-curve phenomenon was not reported in the ABCD trial; however, it is difficult to rely on this information because of the small sample size. No adverse consequence was due to tight control in the ABCD or the UKPDS; this should allay any fear of the J-curve phenomenon in diabetic, hypertensive patients.

The HOT study [52] was the largest, randomized, actively-controlled trial and 8% of participants were diabetics. BP was reduced from 170/105 mm Hg to 140/81 mm Hg in the group whose BP was controlled most intensively and was followed for most than 3.8 years. There were trends of benefit in all outcome categories (see Table 4). In a subgroup analysis of diabetic patients, the most significant differences were reduction of major CV events and CV mortality in target group who had diastolic BP $\leq$ 80 mm Hg. The main reason for the reported benefit in the HOT study is related to the benefits that were observed in the diabetes subgroup; however, the true achieved BP in diabetic patients was not reported in the study. Thus, the results of these three recent RCTs clearly emphasize the importance of aggressive BP control in diabetic, hypertensive patients. Based on the data that are available from these studies, it seems prudent to recommend the target goal for BP to be less than 130/80 mm Hg.

### What should be the target blood pressure in diabetic patients who have renal failure?

JNC VII guidelines recommend that BP should be decreased to 125/75 mm Hg in patients who have proteinuria in excess of 1 g/d, primarily based on the RCT, Modification of Diet in Renal Disease Study [76,77]. Diabetic patients who required insulin were excluded from this study and diabetics accounted for only 3% of study subjects. Nevertheless, because renal dysfunction is related clearly to the BP values, it seems reasonable to recommend the target BP of 125/75 mm Hg in diabetic patients who have renal insufficiency.

## Combination therapy

### Rationale for combination therapy

For diabetic patients who have moderate or severe hypertension, two or more antihypertensive agents often are required to control the BP. In the UKPDS, 62% of subjects needed two agents and 29% of patients in the tight control group needed more than two agents to achieve a BP that was less than 150/85 mm Hg [3]. The combination therapy has the following potential advantages: (1) synergistic or additive effect in decreasing BP because each drug has different modes of actions; (2) neutralizes the side effects; (3) less dosage-dependent adverse effects because of lower dosages of each agent; and (4) better compliance with combination pills, but at a higher price (see Table 2). For example, the hypokalemic effect of thiazide or loop diuretics can be neutralized by potassium-sparing diuretics, ACE inhibitors, and ARBs. The compensatory activation of renin and

Table 6
Randomized, controlled trials of combination therapy versus monotherapy for hypertension in patients who had type 2 diabetes

| Group 1 | Group 2 | BP control | Reference |
|---|---|---|---|
| HCTZ | HCTZ + fosinopril | G2 > G1[a] | Plat & Saini, 1997 [80] |
| Bendrofluazide | bendrofluazide + atenolol | G2 > G1 | Corcoran et al, 1987 [81] |
| Bendrofluazide | bendrofluazide + nifedipine | G2 > G1 | Corcoran et al, 1987 [81] |
| Bendrofluazide | bendrofluazide + captopril | G2 > G1 | Corcoran et al, 1987 [81] |
| ACE inhibitor | ACE inhibitor + amlodipine | G2 > G1 | Shigihara et al, 2000 [82] |
| Lisinopril | Lisinopril + candesartan | G2 > G1 | Mogensen et al, 2000 [64] |
| Candesartan | Lisinopril + candesartan | G2 > G1 | Mogensen et al, 2000 [64] |

[a] BP control was more effective in group 2 than in group 1.

angiotensin II system by diuretics can be counteracted by ACE inhibitors or ARBs. Dose-dependent ankle edema from CCBs is less frequent with the addition of diuretics [78] or ACE inhibitors [55] because of the lower dosage requirements of CCBs. The adverse effects of CCBs (eg, headache, flushing, ankle edema) and ACE inhibitors (eg, cough) are less frequent when low dosages of CCBs were combined with small dosages of ACE inhibitor therapy [55,79].

*Monotherapy versus combination therapy in diabetic patients*

The long-term outcomes that compare different combination regimens have not been vigorously tested in RCTs in the general or diabetic population. Studies with short-term efficacy evaluation of combination therapy versus monotherapy in diabetic patients also are limited (Table 6). A recent study compared the effects of fosinopril, 20 mg, plus hydrochlorothiazide (HCTZ), 12.5 mg, with HCTZ, 25 mg, in 160 hypertensive, diabetic patients [80]. The combination therapy showed better BP control and less metabolic disturbance in potassium, lipid, and glucose homeostasis. Another study enrolled hypertensive, patients who had type 2 diabetes and

microalbuminuria. ACE inhibitors plus amlodipine was more effective in decreasing BP and reducing proteinuria than ACE inhibitors alone [82]. In another study of 37 patients who had clinical diabetic nephropathy, when the BP level was controlled to the same extent in both groups (trandolapril versus trandolapril plus verapamil), the group who received combination therapy showed a better antiproteinuric effect [83]. The comparison of candesartan, lisinopril, or the combination of both on BP and urinary albumin excretion was conducted in 199 patients who had type 2 diabetes, microalbuminuria, and hypertension in an RCT [64]. The combination regimen was more effective in decreasing BP and reducing proteinuria than either agent alone.

*Comparison of various combination therapies in diabetic patients*

Two or more antihypertensive agents were combined to control the BP in a significant proportion of patients in most long-term RCTs (see Tables 3–5). Because of the original study designs it is difficult to further analyze and compare the effects of different combination regimens in those trials. Trials that compared the effectiveness of BP control with different antihypertensive

Table 7
Comparison of different combination therapies for hypertension in patients who had type 2 diabetes in randomized, controlled trials

| Group 1 | Group 2 | BP control | Reference |
|---|---|---|---|
| HCTZ + captopril | Nifedipine + captopril | NS[a] | Souviron Rodriguez et al, 1992 [84] |
| Bendrofluazide + nifedipine | Bendrofluazide + atenolol | NS | Corcoran et al, 1987 [81] |
| Bendrofluazide + nifedipine | Bendrofluazide + captopril | NS | Corcoran et al, 1987 [81] |
| Bendrofluazide + atenolol | Bendrofluazide + captopril | NS | Corcoran et al, 1987 [81] |
| Chlortalidone + atenolol | Trandolapril + verapamil | NS | Schneider et al, 1996 [85] |

[a] NS: There were no significant differences in BP control between group 1 and group 2.

combinations in diabetic patients are limited (Table 7). In a small study, 37 diabetic patients who failed captopril monotherapy were randomized to HCTZ or nifedipine and the study continued for 4 months [84]. There was a statistically insignificant trend which showed that captopril plus HCTZ was more effective in controlling BP than captopril plus nifedipine without changes in plasma glucose, cholesterol, triglycerides, HDL-cholesterol, or uric acid [84]. In a diuretic-based study, 25 type 2 diabetics who remained hypertensive after TD therapy were randomized in a crossover design, in which atenolol or slow-release nifedipine or captopril was added [81]. All three combinations were more effective than thiazide alone and there was no significant difference in BP controls 15 hours after administration of the evening dosage. The combination of ACE inhibitors and CCBs has been advocated for BP control in diabetic patients because of its potentially better antiproteinuric efficacy [86]; however, there is no convincing evidence that this combination is more effective. For example, in a small study, 24 type 2 diabetics who had hypertension were assigned randomly to combined slow-release verapamil plus trandolapril or to atenolol plus chlortalidone. There was no difference in BP control after 12 weeks of follow-up between the two combination groups [85].

## Summary

Large, placebo-controlled RCTs that involve only diabetic patients who have hypertension have not been performed. Subgroup analyses of hypertension control from several recent RCTs unequivocally demonstrated greater benefit in diabetic populations (see Table 3) with ACE inhibitors, TDs, and CCBs. Treatment with βBs (atenolol) also was beneficial in diabetic patients who had hypertension in the actively-controlled UKPDS [5]. The results of three RCTs support intensive BP control in diabetic patients (see Table 4). In these trials, diabetic patients gained more benefit than nondiabetic patients [14,30,40]. Such an effect is consistent with the fact that diabetics are at higher risk for CV events [10,87,88]. Although there are limited data from RCTs with head-to-head comparison of newer agents (eg, ACE inhibitors, ARBs, CCBs) to show that these drugs are better than diuretics and βBs in reducing CV events by treating hypertension in the diabetic population, the available data support ACE

inhibitors (and ARBs if ACE inhibitors are not tolerated) as an initial drug of choice in diabetic, hypertensive patients (see Table 5) [53,54]. Most diabetic patients require three or four drugs to control their BP to target range; as such, it is not necessary to justify the choice of any single class of drug.

Tight BP control is cost-effective and is more rewarding than hyperglycemic control in diabetic, hypertensive patients. The optimal goal in diabetics should be to achieve BP that is less than 130/80 mm Hg. Appropriate action should be taken if BP is greater than 140/85 mm Hg. In subjects who have diabetes and renal insufficiency, the BP should be decreased to less than 125/75 mm Hg to delay the progression of renal failure. Limited data suggest that an ACE inhibitor or an ARB is the agent of choice, especially in patients who have proteinuria or renal insufficiency. βBs can be the first-line agent in diabetics who have CAD. TDs and CCBs are the second line drugs. AAAs should be avoided. Most hypertensive patients require more than one agent to adequately control their BP. There is no evidence to support one combination regimen over the others, nevertheless, the combination of an ACE inhibitor with a TD or a βB may be more beneficial and cost effective than other combinations in the diabetic population. Large outcome studies that compare different combination therapies in hypertensive, diabetic patients are needed.

## References

[1] Herlitz J. How to improve the cardiac prognosis for diabetes. Diabetes Care 1999;22(Suppl 2):B89–96.
[2] Fagan TC, Deedwania PC. The cardiovascular dysmetabolic syndrome. Am J Med 1998;105(1A):77S–82S.
[3] UK Prospective Diabetes Study Group. Tight blood pressure control and risk of macrovascular and microvascular complications in type 2 diabetes: UKPDS 38. BMJ 1998;317:703–13.
[4] UK Prospective Diabetes Study Group. Intensive blood-glucose control with sulphonylureas or insulin compared with conventional treatment and risk of complications in patients with type 2 diabetes (UKPDS 33). Lancet 1998;352:837–53.
[5] UK Prospective Diabetes Study Group. Efficacy of atenolol and captopril in reducing risk of both macrovascular and microvascular complications in type 2 diabetes (UKPDS 39). BMJ 1998;317:713–20.
[6] Haffner SM. Epidemiology of type 2 diabetes: risk factors. Diabetes Care 1998;21(Suppl 3):C3–6.

[7] Tarnow L, Rossing P, Gall M-A, et al. Prevalence of arterial hypertension in diabetic patients before and after the JNC-V. Diabetes Care 1994;17:1247–51.

[8] Hypertension in diabetes study (HDS). I. Prevalence of hypertension in newly presenting type 2 diabetic patients and the association with risk factors for cardiovascular and diabetic complications. J Hypertension 1993;11:309–17.

[9] Burt VL, Whelton P, Roccella EJ, et al. Prevalence of hypertension in the US adult population. Results from the Third National Health and Nutrition Examination Survey, 1988–91. Hypertension 1995; 25:305–13.

[10] DeStafano F, Ford ES, Newman J, Stevenson JM, Wetterhall SF, Anda RF, et al. Risk factors for coronary heart disease mortality among persons with diabetes. Ann Epidemiol 1993;3:27–34.

[11] Criqui MH. Epidemiology of atherosclerosis: an updated overview. Am J Cardiol 1986;57:18C–23C.

[12] Wilson PW. An epidemiologic perspective of systemic hypertension, ischemic heart disease, and heart failure. Framingham Heart Study. Am J Cardiol 1997;80(9B):3J–8J.

[13] The National High Blood Pressure Education Program Working Group. National High Blood Pressure Education Program Working Group report on hypertension in diabetes. Hypertension 1994;23: 145–58.

[14] Systolic hypertension in Europe trial investigators. Effects of calcium-channel blockade in older patients with diabetes and systolic hypertension. N Engl J Med 1999;340:677–84.

[15] Ritz E, Rychlik I, Locatelli F, Halimi S. End-stage renal failure in type 2 diabetes: a medical catastrophe of worldwide dimensions. Am J Kidney Dis 1999; 34:795–808.

[16] Cost effectiveness of intensive treatment of hypertension. Based on presentations by Donald S. Shepard, PhD and Dominic Hodgkin, PhD. Am J Manag Care 1998;4(12 Suppl):S765–9 [discussion S770].

[17] UK Prospective Diabetes Study Group. Cost effectiveness analysis of improved blood pressure control in hypertensive patients with type 2 diabetes: UKPDS 40. BMJ 1998;12;317(7160):720–6.

[18] Elliott WJ, Weir DR, Black HR. Cost-effectiveness of the lower treatment goal (of JNC VI) for diabetic hypertensive patients. Joint National Committee on Prevention, Detection, Evaluation, and Treatment of High Blood Pressure. Arch Intern Med 2000;8; 160(9):1277–83.

[19] The Sixth Report of The Joint National Committee on Prevention Detection, Evaluation, and Treatment of High Blood Pressure. Arch Intern Med 1997;157:2413–46.

[20] Prencipe M, Casini AR, Santini M, Ferretti C, Scaldaferri N, Culasso F. Prevalence, awareness, treatment and control of hypertension in the elderly: results from a population survey. J Hum Hypertens 2000;14:825–30.

[21] Kjeldsen SE, Dahlof B, Devereux RB, Julius S, de Faire U, Fyhrquist F, et al. Lowering of blood pressure and predictors of response in patients with left ventricular hypertrophy: the LIFE study. Losartan Intervention For Endpoint. Am J Hypertens 2000;13:899–906.

[22] American Diabetes Association. Position statement: treatment of hypertension in adults with diabetes. 2002;25:571–3.

[23] 1999 Canadian recommendations for the management of hypertension. CMAJ 1999;161(12 Suppl): S1–17.

[24] Gainer JV, Morrow JD, Loveland A, King DJ, Brown NJ. Effect of bradykinin-receptor blockade on the response to angiotensin-converting-enzyme inhibitor in normotensive and hypertensive subjects. N Engl J Med 1998;339:1285–92.

[25] Wright JM. Choosing a first-line drug in the management of elevated blood pressure: what is the evidence? 2: Beta-blockers. CMAJ 2000;163(2):188–92.

[26] Hansson L, Lindholm LH, Niskanen L, Lanke J, Hendner T, et al. Effect of angiotensin-converting-enzyme inhibition compared with conventional therapy on cardiovascular morbidity and mortality in hypertension: the Captopril Prevention Project (CAPPP) randomized trial. Lancet 1999;353:611–6.

[27] The Heart Outcomes Prevention Evaluation Study Investigators. Effects of angiotensin-converting-enzyme inhibitor, ramipril, on cardiovascular events in high-risk patients. N Engl J Med 2000;342: 145–53.

[28] Galletti F, Strazzullo P, Capaldo B, Carretta R, Fabris F, Ferrara LA, et al. Controlled study of the effect of angiotensin converting enzyme inhibition versus calcium-entry blockade on insulin sensitivity in overweight hypertensive patients: Trandolapril Italian Study (TRIS). J Hypertens 1999;17:439–45.

[29] Buller GK, Perazella M. ACE inhibitor-induced hypoglycaemia. Am J Med 1991;91:104–5.

[30] Heart Outcomes Prevention Evaluation (HOPE) study Investigators. Effects of ramipril on cardiovascular and microvascular outcomes in people with diabetes mellitus: results of the HOPE study and MICRO-HOPE substudy. Lancet 2000; 355:253–9.

[31] Reardon LC, Macpherson DS. Hyperkalemia in outpatients using angiotensin-converting enzyme inhibitors. How much should we worry? Arch Intern Med 1998;12;158(1):26–32.

[32] Goodfriend TL, Elliott ME, Catt KJ. Drug therapy: angiotensin receptors and their antagonists. N Engl J Med 1996;334:1649–54.

[33] Wright JM. Choosing a first-line drug in the management of elevated blood pressure: what is the evidence? 3: Angiotensin-converting-enzyme, ACE inhibitors. CMAJ 2000;163:293–6.

[34] Piepho RW. Overview of the angiotensin-converting-enzyme inhibitors. Am J Health Syst Pharm 2001;57(Suppl 1):S3–7.

[35] Warner KK, Visconti JA, Tschampel MM. Angiotensin II receptor blockers in patients with ACE inhibitor-induced angioedema. Ann Pharmacother 2000;34:526–8.

[36] Grossman E. Angiotensin II receptor blockers. Arch Intern Med 2000;160:1905–11.

[37] Bakris GL, Siomos M, Richardson D, Janssen I, Bolton WK, Hebert L, et al. ACE inhibition or angiotensin receptor blockade: impact on potassium in renal failure. Kidney Int 2000;58:2084–92.

[38] Shah S, Khatri I, Freis ED. Mechanism of antihypertensive effect of thiazide diuretics. Am Heart J 1978;95(5):611–8.

[39] Weidmann PO, Boehlen L, de Courten M. Pathogenesis and treatment of hypertension associated with diabetes mellitus. Am Heart J 1993;125:1498–513.

[40] Systolic Hypertension in the Elderly Program Cooperative Research Group. Effect of diuretic-based antihypertensive treatment on cardiovascular disease risk in older diabetic patients with isolated systolic hypertension. JAMA 1996;276:1886–92.

[41] Kostis JB, Berge KG, Davis BR, Hawkins CM, Probstfield J. Effect of atenolol and reserpine on selected events in the systolic hypertension in the elderly program (SHEP). Am J Hypertens 1995; 8(12 Pt 1):1147–53.

[42] Warram J, Laffel LM, Valsania P, et al. Excess mortality associated with diuretic therapy in diabetes mellitus. Arch Intern Med 1991;151:1350–6.

[43] David S, Siscovick TE, Raghunathan BM, Psaty TD, Koepsell KG, Wicklund XL, et al. Diuretic Therapy for Hypertension and the Risk of Primary Cardiac Arrest. N Engl J Med 1994; 330:1852–7.

[44] Zuanetti G, Latini R. Impact of pharmacological treatment on mortality after myocardial infarction in diabetic patients. J Diabet Complications 1997; 11:131–6.

[45] Gress TW, Nieto J, Shahar I, Brancati FL. Hypertension and antihypertensive therapy as risk factors for type 2 diabetes mellitus. For the atherosclerosis risk in communities study. N Engl J Med 2000;342: 905–12.

[46] Veterans Administration Cooperative Study Group on Antihypertensive Agents. Propranolol or hydrochlorothiazide alone for the initial treatment of hypertension. IV. Effect on plasma glucose and glucose tolerance. Hypertension 1985;7:1008–16.

[47] Ravid M, Brosh D, Levi Z, Bar-Dayan Y, et al. Use of enalapril to attenuate decline in renal function in normotensive, normoalbuminuric patients with type 2 diabetes mellitus. A randomized, controlled trial. Ann Intern Med 1998;128:982–8.

[48] Deacon SP, Barnett D. Comparison of atenolol and propranolol during insulin-induced hypoglycaemia. BMJ 1976;2:272–3.

[49] Kerr D, Macdonald IA, Heller SR, et al. Beta-adrenoceptor blockade and hypoglycaema. Br J Clin Pharmacol 1990;29:685–93.

[50] Hirsch IB, Boyle PJ, Craft S, Cryer PE. Higher glycemic thresholds for symptoms during beta-adrenergic blockade in IDDM. Diabetes 1991; 40(9):1177–86.

[51] Lyngsoe J, Sorensen M, Sjostrand H, et al. The effect of sustained release verapamil on glucose metabolism in patients with NIDDM. Drugs 1992;1: 85–7.

[52] Hansson L, Zanchetti A, Carruthers SG, et al. Effects of intensive blood pressure lowering and low dose aspirin in patients with hypertension: principal results of the Hypertension Optimal Treatment (HOT) randomized trial. Lancet 1998;351:1755–62.

[53] Estacio RO, Jeffers BW, Hiatt WR, et al. The effect of nisoldipine as compared with enalapril on cardiovascular outcomes in patients with non-insulin dependent diabetes and hypertension. N Engl J Med 1998;338:645–52.

[54] Tatti P, Pahor M, Byington R. Outcome results of the fosinopril versus amlodipine cardiovascular events randomized trial (FACET) in patients with hypertension and NIDDM. Diabetes Care 1998;21: 597–603.

[55] Messerli FH, Oparil S, Feng Z. Comparison of efficacy and side effects of combination therapy of angiotensin-converting enzyme inhibitor (benazepril) with calcium antagonist (either nifedipine or amlodipine) versus high-dose calcium antagonist monotherapy for systemic hypertension. Am J Cardiol 2000;86:1182–7.

[56] Lithell HO. Hyperinsulinemia, insulin resistance, and the treatment of hypertension. Am J Hypertens 1996;9:150S–4S.

[57] Andersen P, Seljeflot I, Herzog A. Effects of doxazosin and atenolol on atherothrombogenic risk profile in hypertensive middle-age men. J Cardiovasc Pharmacol 1998;31:677–83.

[58] The ALLHAT officers and coordinators for the ALLHAT Collaborative Research Group. The antihypertensive and lipid-lowering treatment to prevent heart attack trial (ALLHAT). Major cardiovascular events in hypertensive patients randomized to doxazosin vs. chlorthalidone. JAMA 2000;283:1967–75.

[59] Bauer JH, Jones LB, Gaddy P. Effects of prazosin therapy on blood pressure, renal function, and body fluid composition. Arch Intern Med 1984;114: 1196–200.

[60] Leenen FHH, Smith DL, Faraks RM, Reeves RA, Marquez-Julio A. Vasodilators and regression of left ventricular hypertrophy: hydralazine versus prazosin in hypertensive patients. Am J Med 1987;82: 969–78.

[61] Liebson PR, Grandits GA, Dianzumba S. Comparison of 5 antihypertensive monotherapies and placebo for change in left ventricular mass in patients receiving nutritional-hygienic therapy in the treatment of mild hypertension study. Circulation 1995; 91:698–706.

[62] Gottdiener JS, Reda DJ, Massie BM. Effect of single-drug therapy on reduction of left ventricular mass in mild to moderate hypertension: comparison of six antihypertensive agents. Circulation 1997;95: 2007–14.

[63] Liao Y, Husain A. The chymase-angiotensin system in humans: biochemistry, molecular biology and potential role in cardiovascular diseases. Can J Cardiol 1995;11(Suppl F):13F–9F.

[64] Mogensen CE, Neldam S, Tikkanen I, Oren S, Viskoper R, Watts RW, et al. Randomised controlled trial of dual blockade of renin-angiotensin system in patients with hypertension, microalbuminuria, and non-insulin dependent diabetes: the candesartan and lisinopril microalbuminuria (CALM) study. BMJ 2000;321(7274):1440–4.

[65] Lacourciere Y, Belanger A, Godin C, Halle JP, Ross S, Wright N, et al. Long-term comparison of losartan and enalapril on kidney function in hypertensive type 2 diabetics with early nephropathy. Kidney Int 2000;58(2):762–9.

[66] Pohl M, Cooper M, Ulrey J, Pauls J, Rohse R. Safety and efficacy of irbesartan in hypertensive patients with type 2 diabetes and proteinuria [abstract]. Am J Hypertens 1997;10:105A.

[67] Lindholm LH, Hansson L, Ekbom T, Dahlof B, Lanke J, Linjer E, et al. Comparison of antihypertensive treatments in preventing cardiovascular events in elderly diabetic patients: results from the Swedish Trial in Old Patients with Hypertension-2. STOP Hypertension-2 Study Group. J Hypertens 2000;18(11):1671–5.

[68] Hansson L, Lindholm LH, Ekbom T, Dahlöf B, Lanke J, Scherstén B, et al, for the STOP-Hypertension-2 study group. Randomised trial of old and new antihypertensive drugs in elderly patients: cardiovascular mortality and morbidity in the Swedish Trial in Old Patients with Hypertension-2 study. Lancet 1999;354:1751–6.

[69] Hansson L, Hedner T, Lund-Johansen P, Kjeldsen SE, Lindholm LH, Syvertsen JO, et al, for the NORDIL Study Group. Randomised trial of effects of calcium antagonists compared with diuretics and β-blockers on cardiovascular morbidity and mortality in hypertension: the Nordic Diltiazem (NORDIL) study. Lancet 2000;356:359–65.

[70] Brown MJ, Palmer CR, Castaigne A, de Leeuw PW, Mancia G, Rosenthal T, et al. Morbidity and mortality in patients randomized to double-blind treatment with a long-acting calcium-channel blocker or diuretic in the International Nifedipine GITS study: Intervention as a Goal in Hypertension Treatment (INSIGHT). Lancet 2000;356:366–72.

[71] Lewis EJ, Hunsicker LG, Bain RP, Rohde RD. The effect of angiotensin-converting-enzyme inhibition on diabetic nephropathy. N Engl J Med 1993;329: 1456–62.

[72] Ravid M, Broth D, Levi Z, Bar-Dayan Y, et al. Use of enalapril to attenuate decline in renal function in normotensive, normoalbuminuric patients with type 2 diabetes mellitus. A randomized, controlled trial. Ann Intern Med 1998;128:982–8.

[73] Mogensen CE. Renoprotective role of ACE inhibitors in diabetic nephropathy. Br Heart J 1994;72(3 Suppl):S38–45.

[74] Ruddy M. Angiotensin II receptor blockade in diabetic nephropathy. Am J Hypertens 2002;15:466.

[75] Estacio RO, Jeffers BW, Gifford N, Dchrier RW. Effect of blood pressure control on diabetic microvascular complications in patients with hypertension and type 2 diabetes. Diabetes Care 2000;23(Suppl 2): B54–64.

[76] Peterson JC, Adler S, Burkart JM, et al. Blood pressure control, proteinuria, and the progression of renal disease: the Modification of Diet in Renal Disease Study. Ann Intern Med 1995;123:754–62.

[77] Lazarus JM, Bourgoignie JJ, Buckalew VM, et al, for the Modification of Diet in Renal Disease Study Group. Achievement and safety of low blood pressure goal in chronic renal disease: the Modification of Diet in Renal Disease Study Group. Hypertension 1997;29:641–50.

[78] Luscher TF, Waeber B. Efficacy and safety of various combination therapies based on a calcium antagonist in essential hypertension: results of a placebo-controlled randomized trial. J Cardiovasc Pharmacol 1993;21(2):305–9.

[79] Pittrow DB, Antlsperger A, Welzel D, Wambach G, Schardt W, Weidinger G. Evaluation of the efficacy and tolerability of a low-dose combination of isradipine and spirapril in the first-line treatment of mild to moderate essential hypertension. Cardiovasc Drugs Ther 1997;11(5):619–27.

[80] Plat F, Saini R. Management of hypertension: the role of combination therapy. Am J Hypertens 1997;10(10 Pt 2):262S–71S.

[81] Corcoran JS, Perkins JE, Hoffbrand BI, Yudkin JS. Treating hypertension in non-insulin-dependent diabetes: a comparison of atenolol, nifedipine, and captopril combined with bendrofluazide. Diabet Med 1987;4(2):164–8.

[82] Shigihara T, Sato A, Hayashi K, Saruta T. Effect of combination therapy of angiotensin-converting enzyme inhibitor plus calcium channel blocker on urinary albumin excretion in hypertensive microalbuminuric patients with type II diabetes. Hypertens Res 2000;23(3):219–26.

[83] Bakris GL, Weir MR, DeQuattro V, McMahon FG. Effects of an ACE inhibitor/calcium antagonist combination on proteinuria in diabetic nephropathy. Kidney Int 1998;54(4):1283–9.

[84] Souviron Rodriguez A, Martinez Morillo M. Captopril + hydrochlorothiazide versus captopril + nifedipine in the treatment of arterial hypertension in diabetes mellitus type II [abstract]. Rev Esp Cardiol 1992;45(7):432–7 [in Spanish].

[85] Schneider M, Lerch M, Papiri M, Buechel P, Boehlen L, Shaw S, et al. Metabolic neutrality of

combined verapamil-trandolapril treatment in contrast to beta-blocker-low-dose chlortali done treatment in hypertensive type 2 diabetes. J Hypertens 1993;14(5):669–77.

[86] Sheinfeld GR, Bakris GL. Benefits of combination angiotensin-converting enzyme inhibitor and calcium antagonist therapy for diabetic patients. Am J Hypertens 1999;12(8)(Pt 2):80S–5S.

[87] Stamler J, Vaccaro O, Neaton JD, Wentworth D. Diabetes, other risk factors, and 12-year cardiovascular mortality for men screened in the multiple risk factor intervention trial. Diabetes Care 1993; 16:434–44.

[88] Sniderman A, Michel C, Racine N. Heart disease in patients with diabetes mellitus. J Clin Epidemiol 1992;45:1357–70.

# The Role of Lipid Management in Diabetes

## Om P. Ganda, MD*

*Joslin Diabetes Center, Department of Medicine, Harvard Medical School,
One Joslin Place, # 242, Boston, MA 02115, USA
Department of Endocrinology and Metabolism, Beth-Israel Deaconess Medical Center,
330 Brookline Avenue, Boston, MA 02215, USA*

### Diabetes as a coronary heart disease risk-equivalent

Based on the observations from several epidemiologic studies, diabetes is designated a coronary heart disease (CHD)-risk equivalent by the National Cholesterol Education Program's Adult Treatment Panel III (ATPIII) [1]. The 10-year risk of major CHD events in patients who have diabetes is greater than 20%; this is comparable to the rates that are observed in nondiabetic patients who have established CHD. This inference has been borne out, particularly by data from a population study in Finland [2] and a multi-national study, the Organization to Assess Strategies for Ischemic Syndromes [3], of patients who had type 2 diabetes who frequently had multiple, coexisting risk factors for cardiovascular disease (CVD). The increased risk for CHD may precede the clinical diagnosis of diabetes by many years. This was documented best in the long-term study of more than 117,000 women in the Nurses' Health Study; nearly 6000 women developed diabetes during 20 years of follow-up. There was an approximately twofold to threefold increased risk for myocardial infarction (MI) or stroke during the "prediabetes" period, compared with women who remained nondiabetic [4]. In another study, Multiple Risk Factor Intervention Trial, in a large number of men (348,000, of which 5163 had diabetes), the presence of diabetes was associated with a threefold to fourfold increased risk for age-adjusted cardiovascular mortality at comparable levels of cholesterol, blood pressure, and cigarette smoking [5]. This suggests an enhanced susceptibility of diabetic vasculature to the well-established risk factors for CHD.

### Lipoprotein abnormalities associated with diabetes

Diabetes is associated with multiple disturbances in lipoprotein metabolism that are triggered by insulin deficiency, insulin resistance, and hyperglycemia [6,7]. The diabetic dyslipidemia of type 2 diabetes and insulin resistance is characterized several interrelated abnormalities, including triglyceride-rich lipoproteins (very low density lipoprotein [VLDL], intermediate density lipoprotein [IDL], and remnant particles), low high-density lipoprotein (HDL) cholesterol, and small, dense low-density lipoprotein (LDL) particles. There is an increase in the lipid-rich, large VLDL; upregulation of hepatic sterol regulatory element binding protein–1, which stimulates de novo lipid synthesis; and increased availability of free fatty acids, all of which probably are linked with insulin resistance [7]. The activity of lipoprotein lipase is suppressed which leads to reduced catabolism of triglyceride-rich particles, whereas hepatic lipase activity is increased which facilitates the compositional changes in LDL and HDL particles. Moreover, there is enhanced activity of cholesterol-ester transfer protein which mediates the transfer of triglyceride to LDL and HDL while cholesterol-esters from the latter are shunted to the larger triglyceride-rich particles. Thus, hypertriglyceridemia is linked indirectly with changes in the HDL and LDL composition and associated with increased atherogenesis. The small, dense LDL

* Joslin Diabetes Center. One Joslin Place, # 242
Boston, MA 02215.
*E-mail address:* om.ganda@joslin.harvard.edu
(O.P. Ganda).

particles: (1) bind to intimal proteoglycans more avidly, (2) are more susceptible to oxidation and glycation, and (3) have impaired binding to LDL receptors; all of these factors contribute to the enhanced atherosclerosis in patients who have type 2 diabetes.

In a recent study, lipoprotein particle size and concentrations were characterized by nuclear magnetic resonance in subjects who had type 2 diabetes and normal or impaired insulin sensitivity that was characterized by euglycemic, hyper-insulinemic clamp technique [8]. There was a progressive increase in the size of VLDL particles in patients who were insulin sensitive, insulin resistant, and had type 2 diabetes and a reciprocal decrease in the size of LDL and HDL particles. Conversely, the cholesterol content in large LDL was decreased; the cholesterol content in small LDL was increased in patients who had insulin resistance and type 2 diabetes; and the calculated LDL cholesterol was unchanged, despite increased LDL particle number.

In view of the compositional changes in lipoproteins, the LDL cholesterol that is determined in routine assays tends to underestimate the LDL particle number, particularly in patients who have hypertriglyceridemia [9,10]. Therefore, it was proposed that the direct measurement of apolipoprotein B (apoB) may provide a better estimate of risk in such patients [11]; however, the assays for apoB are not well-standardized and are not widely available. An alternative that was proposed by ATPIII is the calculation of non-HDL cholesterol which estimates the cholesterol content in all atherogenic particles (VLDL, IDL, remnants, LDL, and lipoprotein [LP(a)]). Non-HDL cholesterol was a good predictor for CVD in diabetes according to some population studies, such as the Strong Heart Study [12] and the Hoorn Study [13]. More evidence is needed from intervention trials before drawing definitive conclusions regarding its impact on lipid management. Similarly, whether the determination of postprandial triglyceride levels improves the risk assessment for CHD remains uncertain [14].

## Evidence from lipid lowering trials in diabetes

### Low-density lipoprotein lowering

Given the heterogeneity of lipoprotein and the complexity of lipoprotein metabolism in patients who have diabetes, the optimal approach for lipid management remains to be determined. Over the past 10 years, a variety of randomized, controlled trials with hydroxymethylglutaryl-coenzyme A reductase inhibitors (statins) established the efficacy of these LDL-lowering agents in reducing cardiovascular outcomes. In four of these large trials (Scandinavian Simvastatin Survival Study [4S], Cholesterol and Recurrent Events [CARE], Long-term Intervention with Pravastatin in Ischemic Disease [LIPID], and Air Force/Texas Coronary Atherosclerosis Prevention Study [AF-CAPS/TexCAPS]), subgroup analyses revealed similar coronary artery disease risk reductions in smaller numbers of diabetic patients compared with the general population. (Table 1) [15–21]. The most recent and largest trial (more than 20,000 subjects) was the Heart Protection Study (HPS) which randomized 5963 patients who had diabetes [22,23]. Of these, approximately 2000 had pre-existing CHD; 1000 had other occlusive vascular disease (including cerebrovascular disease), and 3000 had no evidence of CHD or other vascular disease. Noteworthy observations in this 5-year trial in patients who had diabetes were (Fig. 1):

The proportional reductions in clinical CVD events with simvastatin, 40 mg, daily were approximately 25% in each of the categories based on age, gender, obesity, duration of diabetes, degree of control by hemoglobin A, C, and lipid parameters at baseline.

The benefits in the 2592 patients who were older than 65 years were similar to those that were seen in the 3371 patients who were younger than 65 years. This was in contrast to the results in the Pravastatin in Elderly Individuals at Risk of Vascular Disease Trial which was performed in an elderly population (aged 70–82 years at baseline) in which the diabetic subgroup (n = 390) did not achieve a reduction in the major CVD end points over a mean follow-up of 3.2 years [24].

The risk reduction in 2426 subjects who had baseline LDL that was less than 116 mg/dL (3mM) was 27%, similar to those whose LDL was greater than 116 mg/dL (20%).

Among patients who received placebo, the 5-year rates of first major vascular event ranged from 13% in those who had diabetes alone to 36% in those who had diabetes and vascular disease. This supports the concept that the absolute risk of CVD is determined mainly by underlying pre-existing disease, rather than lipid levels.

Table 1
Major CHD event reductions in long-term trials with HMG-CoA reductase inhibitors (Statins)

| Trail | Drug | Baseline LDL (mg/dL)* | Overall patient population | | | Diabetes sub-group | | |
|---|---|---|---|---|---|---|---|---|
| | | | n | Risk-reduction (%) | P | n | Risk-reduction (%) | P |
| Primary prevention | | | | | | | | |
| AFCAPS/TexCAPS | Lovastatin | 156 | 6605 | 37 | <0.001 | 155 | 43 | NS |
| HPS | Simvastatin | 124 | 7150 | 25 | <0.0001 | 3982 | 26 | <0.0001 |
| CARDS | Atorvastatin | 118 | — | — | — | 2838 | 37 | 0.001 |
| ALLHAT-LLT** | Pravastatin | 146 | 10,355 | 9 | NS | 3638 | 11 | NS |
| ASCOT-LLA | Atorvastatin | 132 | 19,342 | 36 | 0.0005 | 2532 | 16 | NS |
| Secondary prevention | | | | | | | | |
| 4S | Simvastatin | 188 | 4444 | 34 | <0.0001 | 202 | 55 | 0.002 |
| 4S (ADA criteria) | Simvastatin | 187 | — | — | — | 483 | 42 | 0.001 |
| CARE | Pravastatin | 139 | 4159 | 23 | <0.001 | 586 | 25 | 0.05 |
| LIPID | Pravastatin | 150 | 9014 | 24 | <0.001 | 782 | 19 | NS |
| HPS | Simvastatin | 124 | 13,386 | 24 | <0.0001 | 1981 | 15 | <0.05 |

*Abbreviations:* AFCAPS/TexCAPS, Airforce/Texas Coronary Atherosclerosis Prevention Study; HPS, Heart Protection Study; CARDS, Collaborative Atorvastatin Diabetes Study; ALLHAT-LLT, Antihypertensive and Lipid-Lowering to Prevent Heart Attack Trial-Lipid Lowering Trial-Lipid Lowering Treatment; ASCOT-LLA, Anglo-Scandinavian Cardiac Outcomes Trial-Lipid Lowering Arm; 4S, Scandinavian Simvastatin Survival Study; CARE, Cholesterol and Recurrent Events; LIPID, Long-term Intervention with Pravastatin in Ischemic Disease.

* Approximate means.
** 155 of the cohort had pre-existing CHD; LDL data obtained in 5–10% of cohort.

Six hundred and fifteen patients had type 1 diabetes. The mean risk reduction was similar to that in the entire cohort.

In addition to these trials, a recently completed secondary prevention trial, the Greek Atorvastatin and Coronary Heart Disease Evaluation study (GREACE), was designed to target LDL cholesterol with atorvastatin, (10–80 mg/d) [25]. The target level of LDL cholesterol (<100 mg/dL) was reached in 95% of patients (compared with 3% of those who were given "usual" medical care). Of the 1600 patients in this study, 313 had diabetes. There was a 51% and 58% reduction in the major coronary end points in total and diabetes subgroup, respectively, during this 3-year trial.

In two primary prevention trials, statin therapy was evaluated in populations who had high risk, based on hypertension. In the Anglo-Scandinavian Cardiac Outcomes Trial–Lipid Lowering Arm Trial, 2531 of 10,305 patients had diabetes [26]. Atorvastatin, 10 mg/d for 3.3 years resulted in a 36% reduction in nonfatal MI and fatal CHD; however, the difference in the diabetic subgroup was not significant. This could be due to the small number of events in this trial over the shorter length of the study. Similarly, in the Antihypertensive and Lipid-Lowering Treatment to Prevent Heart Attack Trial, the lack of benefit

from pravastatin, 40 mg, in the trial group of 10,355 or the diabetic subgroup of 3638 subjects is less surprising [27]. In this study, the cholesterol level that was achieved was only 9% less than in subjects who were given placebo, mainly as a result of the nonstudy use of statin in the control group.

## The Collaborative Atorvastatin Diabetes Study

A Primary Prevention Trial, Collaborative Atorvastatin Diabetes Study (CARDS), exclusively in patients with type 2 diabetes who had one additional risk factor was recently published [28]. A total of 2838 patients, age range 40–75 years, were randomized to 10 mg atorvastatin versus placebo and followed over a mean period of 3.9 years. In this trial, the mean LDL-cholesterol level was 118 mg/dL, which was reduced by 40% in the drug treated group. The combined primary end-points of acute CHD events, coronary revascularization or stroke were reduced by 37% (P = 0.001), whereas stroke events were reduced by 48%, and total mortality by 27% (P = 0.059). The risk reductions were independent of baseline lipid levels and in post-hoc analyses 743 patients with baseline LDL <100 mg/dL had a 26% reduction in major cardiovascular events, which is consistent with the results in the HPS [25].

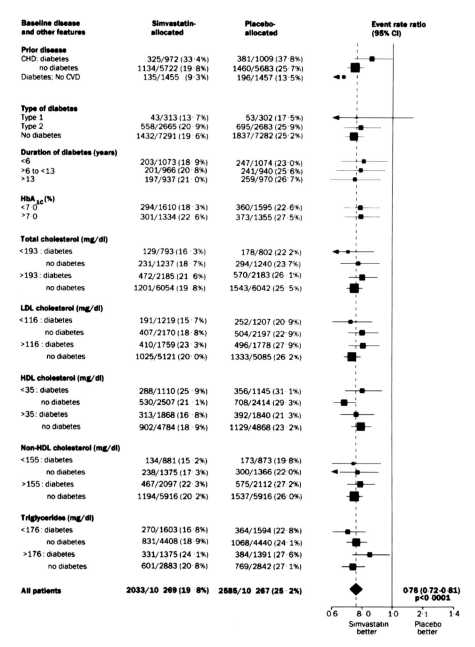

Fig. 1. Effects of simvastatin on first major vascular event in patients who do or do not have diabetes according to presenting features and baseline blood lipid concentrations. CI, confidence interval. The numbers in columns two and three represent the number of individuals with a given characteristic/total number in that group (% of total with the given characteristic). The last column represents the proportional reduction in risk (and CIs); the size of the rectangular box varies according to the relative number of subjects. (*Adapted from* Collins R, Armitage J, Parish S, Sleigh P, Peto R. MRC/BHF Heart Protection Study of cholesterol-lowering with simvastatin in 5963 people with diabetes: a randomised placebo-controlled trial. Lancet 2003;361(9374):2005–16; with permission.)

*Intensive versus moderate lipid intervention in acute coronary syndromes*

Two Large Lipid-Intervention Trials in patients with acute coronary syndromes were recently completed. PROVE-IT (Pravastatin or Atorvastatin Evaluation and Infection Therapy) Trial compared high dose (80 mg) atorvastatin with moderate dose pravastatin (40 mg) in 4162 patients presenting within 10 days of the acute coronary event. The median LDL reduction to 62 mg/dL and 95 mg/dL respectively, resulted in a 16% reduction in the composite primary endpoint ($P = 0.005$) over 24 months [29]. A similar, but non-significant, trend was seen in 734 (18%) of patients with diabetes. There were no major adverse effects except a small but significant difference in the number of patients (3.3% versus 1.1%) with ALT >3 fold above the upper limit of normal. In contrast, in the A to Z trial, 4497 patients presenting with acute coronary syndromes were randomized within 4 days to an early intensive treatment arm with simvastatin 40 mg/d for one month followed by 80 mg/d, and a delayed conservative strategy of placebo for 4 months, followed by 20 mg/d simvastatin [30]. 1059 (24%) of patients had diabetes. There were no significant differences in composite primary end-points in initial 4 months but from 4 thru 24 months, there was a 25% reduction in the simvastatin only group ($P = 0.02$). The differences in outcome between PROVE-IT and the A to Z trial could be due to several possible reasons, including a delayed initiation of intensive treatment and other factors such as less differential in LDL-cholesterol levels, less than expected number of events, and 33% rate of study-drug discontinuation in the A to Z Trial. However, it is noteworthy that, in contrast to the PROVE-IT Trial with 80 mg atorvastatin, there were 9 patients in the 80 mg simvastatin group in the A to Z trial with evidence of myopathy (CK > 10× upper limit of normal) and 3 of these patients had rhabdomyolysis. These findings underscore the need for greater vigilance for adverse effects and safety issues in patients on high dose statins.

The Post Coronary Bypass Graft Trial was an angiographic regression trial that compared aggressive cholesterol lowering with moderate cholesterol lowering. After a mean follow-up of 4.3 years, the angiographic end points were comparable in the subgroup that had diabetes (n = 116) and the nondiabetic cohort (n = 1235) [31].

Thus, the overall efficacy of statins seems to be dependent largely on baseline risk of vascular disease, duration of treatment, and perhaps, the LDL level that is achieved. The ideal level of LDL is unknown; additional trials with specific targets are needed. A recent meta-analysis of 58 randomized trials of cholesterol lowering concluded that an approximate decrease in LDL cholesterol of 40 mg/dL resulted in a 33% decrease in CHD events by 5 years; additional benefits may accrue with a greater decrease in LDL cholesterol over the long term [32]. The average LDL reductions and outcomes seemed to be similar in the diabetic subgroups.

## Triglyceride and high-density lipoprotein intervention

Unlike the plethora of trial evidence of CHD risk reduction with statins, the evidence from drugs to decrease triglycerides or increase HDL cholesterol is sparse. A meta-analysis of 17 observational studies suggested a significant relationship of triglycerides with CHD, even after adjustment for HDL cholesterol, especially in women [33]. In the 4S trial, in post hoc analyses, patients who had the lipid triad (elevated LDL, elevated triglyceride, decreased HDL cholesterol) had the highest event rates in the placebo arm and the greatest risk reduction with simvastatin [34]. Despite a mechanistic plausibility of increased risk with these lipid abnormalities in patients who had metabolic syndrome and diabetes, few long-term randomized trials have been completed (Table 2).

In the Helsinki Heart Study, a primary prevention trial, a small subgroup of 135 patients who had diabetes achieved a 68%, but nonsignificant, decrease in CHD events with gemfibrozil over 5 years [35]. In the St. Mary's Ealing Northwick Park Diabetes Cardiovascular Prevention Study, which included 164 patients who had type 2 diabetes, intervention with bezafibrate resulted in no significant difference in the primary end point of carotid lesions that were detected by ultrasound; however, there were 60% fewer total coronary events over a period of 3 years ($P < 0.01$) [36]. In the Diabetes Atherosclerosis Intervention Study (DAIS), an angiographic regression trial, 418 patients who had type 2 diabetes and evidence of CHD on angiography were treated with fenofibrate or placebo over at least 3 years [37]. The group that received fenofibrate

Table 2
Major cardiovascular trial results with fibrates in patients who have type 2 diabetes

| Trial | Drug | Primary end points | Total subjects/ diabetics | CHD at baseline | Outcome | P value |
|-------|------|--------------------|---------------------------|-----------------|---------|---------|
| HHS | Gemfibrozil | Cardiac events/deaths | 4081/135 | No | CHD reduction: 68% | NS |
| SENDCAP | Bezafibrate | Carotid ultrasound | 164/164 | No | No difference[a] | - |
| DAIS | Fenofibrate | Coronary stenosis on angiography | 418/418 | 48% | Reduced lesion progression | 0.02 |
| VA-HIT | Gemfibrozil | Fatal/nonfatal MI | 2531/627 | Yes | CHD reduction: 24% | <0.05 |

*Abbreviations:* DAIS, Diabetes Atherosclerosis Intervention Study; HHS, Helsinki Heart Study; SENDCAP, St. Mary's Ealing Northwick Park Diabetes Cardiovascular Prevention Study ;VA-HIT, Veterans Administration – HDL Intervention Trial.

[a] 60% fewer coronary events ($P = 0.01$).

showed significantly slower progression of disease and a trend toward fewer clinical end points (38 versus 50) in this small trial.

The largest, randomized clinical trial of fibrate therapy in patients who had diabetes was the Veterans Affairs High-Density Lipoprotein Cholesterol Intervention Trial (VA-HIT) [38]. In this trial, 2531 men who had CHD were recruited who had LDL cholesterol of up to 140 mg/dL; HDL cholesterol that was less than 40 mg/dL, and triglycerides that were up to 300 mg/dL at baseline. Of these, 627 had type 2 diabetes and an additional 363 had evidence for insulin resistance [39]. Treatment with gemfibrozil for a median duration of 5.1 years resulted in 24% risk reduction in the combined outcome of CHD death, MI, and stroke, despite no change in LDL cholesterol; HDL cholesterol increased by 6% and triglyceride levels decreased by 30%. The diabetic subgroup had a greater reduction in the combined end points (32%) compared with the nondiabetics (18%), although these differences were not statistically significant (Fig. 2) [39]. Subsequent analyses from the VA-HIT revealed that the outcomes were not explained by the change in triglycerides and were explained only partially by the increase in HDL cholesterol [40]. The 5-year event rates were correlated highly with insulin resistance [41], with or without diabetes. The event reduction was significantly greater in those who had insulin resistance and was independent of the HDL cholesterol or triglyceride levels, before or after treatment [41]. These analyses suggest the possibility that other antiatherogenic effects of fibrates that are mediated by a variety of mechanisms (eg, PPAR-α agonism, anti-inflammatory effects on vessel wall, fibrinolysis) may contribute to the event reductions that were seen in the VA-HIT.

## Lipid goals in patients who have diabetes

Diabetes is a CHD-risk equivalent, as defined by the ATPIII recommendations. Based on the evidence from the LDL-lowering clinical trials that were summarized above, most patients who have diabetes should have an LDL goal of less than 100 mg/dL (Table 3). If LDL is grater than 130 mg/dL, treatment with LDL-lowering drugs should be initiated simultaneously with therapeutic lifestyle changes (TLC) to achieve the LDL goal [1]. The American Diabetes Association (ADA) has the same recommendations for LDL goal [42]. In addition, the ADA recommends a triglyceride goal of less than 150 mg/dL and an HDL cholesterol goal of greater than 40 mg/dL in men and greater than 50 mg/dL in women (see Table 3). According to ATPIII, however, when triglyceride levels are elevated (200–499 mg/dL) after achieving LDL goal, non-HDL cholesterol should be the secondary target of therapy. No HDL goal is specified in ATPIII because of the lack of sufficient evidence. It is recommended that if HDL remains low after LDL and non-HDL goals are achieved or if triglyceride is less than 200 mg/dL but HDL is low (isolated low HDL cholesterol), drugs for increasing HDL can be considered.

Following the recent evidence from the newer Statin Trials including HPS, ASCOT-LLA, and PROVE-IT, as well as, CARDS summarized earlier, the ATP III panel of the NCEP recently updated their current guidelines [43]. The salient features of this update are depicted in Box 1. It is now recommended that LDL-lowering drug therapy be considered simultaneously with lifestyle changes in high risk patients if LDL exceeds 100 mg/dL. In patients in very high risk category, such as patients with diabetes and CVD, a therapeutic option is to lower LDL-cholesterol goal to <70 mg/dL, regardless of the baseline LDL-cholesterol.

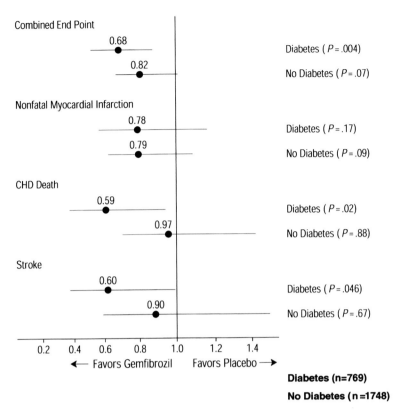

Fig. 2. Hazard ratios for major cardiovascular events with gemfibrozil compared with placebo in patients who do and do not have diabetes. (*From* Rubins HB, Robins SJ, Collins D, Nelson DB, Elam MB, Schaefer EJ, et al. Diabetes, plasma insulin, and cardiovascular disease: subgroup analysis from the Department of Veterans Affairs high-density lipoprotein intervention trial (VA-HIT). Arch Intern Med 2002;162(22):2597–604; with permission.)

Moreover, when LDL-lowering drug therapy is used in high risk patients, the intensity of therapy should be sufficient to achieve at least a 30% to 40% reduction in LDL-cholesterol levels, which correlates roughly to a 30% to 40% reduction in risk for myocardial infarction or CVD mortality [43].

In patients who have triglycerides that are greater than 500 mg/dL and diabetic lipemia (triglycerides higher than 1000 mg/dL), the initial aim is to decrease triglycerides to prevent acute pancreatitis. This requires a combination of a very low fat diet, weight reduction, increased physical activity, and a triglyceride-lowering drug. After triglyceride levels have been lowered to less than 500 mg/dL, the LDL and other lipid targets should be assessed.

**Principles of lipid management in diabetes**

Treatment of lipid disorders that frequently are associated with diabetes, includes TLCs,

optimal glycemic control, and pharmacologic agents. The priorities are decreasing LDL cholesterol and non-HDL cholesterol; these are followed by decreasing triglycerides and increasing HDL, as per recommendations by ATPIII and all diabetes/endocrine organizations. LDL-lowering trials with statins, particularly including the new evidence from the HPS, make a persuasive argument for the efficacy and safety of the statin therapy which is underused in this high-risk population. In highly-motivated individuals, LDL cholesterol reductions of 30%, by dietary approaches (comparable to with statins), were demonstrated [44]. In most patients, however, LDL cholesterol reductions of more than 10% to 15% are not easily achievable with nonpharmacologic approaches. Therefore, the ATPIII recommends simultaneous initiation of statin therapy if LDL cholesterol is greater than 130 mg/dL. The statins provide LDL cholesterol reductions of up to 55% to 60%; the most recently available agent,

Table 3
Categories of risk based on lipid levels (mg/dL) in adults who have diabetes, as defined by the American Diabetes Association

| Risk | LDL cholesterol | HDL cholesterol[a] | Triglycerides |
|---|---|---|---|
| High | >130 | <40 | <400 |
| Borderline | 100–129 | 40–59 | 150–399 |
| Low | <100 | >60 | <150 |

[a] For women, the HDL cholesterol value should be increased by 10 mg/dL.

rosuvastatin, is the most potent (Table 4) [1,45]. The simultaneous adherence to dietary measures, including soluble fiber, soy protein, plant sterols, and weight-management, is essential to maintain the lipid goals with lower dosages of drugs. The effectiveness of statins and other lipid-lowering agents in diabetic patients is comparable to that in nondiabetic patients [46,47].

If LDL cholesterol is 100 mg/dL to 129 mg/dL at baseline or on treatment, therapeutic options include intensifying the LDL-lowering therapy; adding a drug to modify other atherogenic components (fibrate or nicotinic acid), or intensifying control of other risk factors, including hypertension and hyperglycemia. Fibrates or niacin also would be indicated in patients who have hypertriglyceridemia or low HDL cholesterol who already are at or close to LDL goals. In the DAIS trial, fenofibrate retarded the progression of atherosclerosis [37]; in VA-HIT, gemfibrozil therapy was associated with significant reductions in clinical end points [38–40]. The findings of the HPS, however, raise the concern that the level of CHD risk, rather than the baseline LDL level, determines the benefits of further LDL-lowering by statins [22,23]. The US Food and Drug Administration recently revised the consumer package insert for simvastatin based on these results and it recommends consideration of this therapy for all patients who have CHD or diabetes, based on their proven high risk for CVD events.

Nicotinic acid (niacin) is associated with the greatest increase in HDL cholesterol and is considered to be a drug of choice in patients who have low HDL [1,46], particularly in combination therapy with other agents. The principal concern is its tolerability and adherence to higher dosage. Recent multi-center trials showed no significant effects on glycemic control with up to 3 g of crystalline niacin [48] or 1 g to 1.5 g of extended release niacin, niaspan [47,49]. It is the only agent that is effective in lowering LP(a) levels. Recently, the availability of ezitimibe, a cholesterol absorption inhibitor that acts at the site of putative cholesterol transfer in the gut, has expanded the options for LDL lowering [50]. It decreases LDL cholesterol an average of 15% to 20% and the effects are additive to the effect of statins. Thus, the addition of 10 mg of ezitimibe to low-dosage statins decreased LDL cholesterol in an amount that was approximately equivalent to tripling the dosage of the statins [50]. It is well-tolerated and, in this regard, provides an alternative to the poorly-tolerated bile-acid sequestrants.

---

**Box 1.  Update of NCEP-ATPIII Recommendations for LDL-C in High Risk Persons**

- LDL-C goal of <70 mg/dL is a therapeutic option on the basis of clinical trial evidence, especially in very high risk patients.
- If LDL-C >100 mg/dL, LDL-lowering drug is indicated simultaneously with therapeutic lifestyle changes.
- If baseline LDL-C is <100 mg/dL, drug treatment to reach an LDL-C <70 mg/dL is a therapeutic option based on clinical trial evidence.
- When LDL-lowering drug therapy is employed in high-risk or moderatively high risk persons, It is advised that the intensity of therapy be sufficient to achieve at least a 305-405 reduction in LDL-C levels.
- In high risk person with high TGL or Low HDL, consider combination treatment using a fibrate or nicotinic acid plus LDL-lowering drug.
- If TGL >200 mg/dL, non-HDL-C (total C minus HDL) is a secondary target of therapy with a goal of 30 mg/dL higher than the LDL goal.

Table 4
The range of the lipid effects of commonly used drugs

| Drug | LDL cholesterol (%) | HDL cholesterol (%) | Triglycerides (%) |
|------|---------------------|---------------------|-------------------|
| Statins | −18 to −55 | +5 to +15 | −7 to −30 |
| Fibrates | −5 to −20* | +10 to +20 | −20 to −50 |
| Niacin | −5 to −25 | +15 to +35 | −20 to −50 |
| Bile acid sequestrants | −15 to −30 | +3 to +5 | No change or increase |
| Ezetimibe | −15 to −20 | +1 to +2 | −5 to −10 |

*, may increase in patients with high triglycerides.

*Adapted from* Executive summary of the Third Report of the National Cholesterol Education Program (NCEP) Expert Panel on Detection, Evaluation, and Treatment of High Blood Cholesterol in adults (Adult Treatment Panel III). JAMA 2001;285(19):2486–97, with permission; and Gagne C, Bays HE, Weiss SR, Mata P, Quinto K, Melino M, et al. Efficacy and safety of ezetimibe added to ongoing statin therapy for treatment of patients with primary hypercholesterolemia. Am J Cardiol 2002;90(10):1084–91; with permission.

## Role of combination therapy in diabetes and dyslipidemia

Despite the known pharmacologic effects of fibrates and nicotinic acid in ameliorating the underlying defects of diabetic dyslipidemia (increased triglyceride-rich lipoproteins; low HDL cholesterol; small, dense LDL particles), the role of combining these agents with statins remains uncertain and further clinical trials are needed. Trials like the VA-HIT and DAIS are supportive of the potential of adding fibrates to statins because combined lipid disorders are common in patients who have insulin resistance and type 2 diabetes. In short-term studies, statins and fibrates were more effective in normalizing all lipid abnormalities than either agent alone without significant risk for adverse events, including myositis [51,52]. Caution should be exercised in patients who have potential drug interactions (eg, cyclosporin, antifungal agents, protease inhibitors, erythromycin) or renal disease. Long-term trials of combination therapy with statins and fenofibrate are in progress (Table 5).

In a study of 160 patients who had CHD and low HDL cholesterol (HDL-Atherosclerosis Treatment Study), combining niacin with somvastatin over a 3-year period in one trial resulted in an impressive reduction in angiographic progression of lesions and clinical end points. A subgroup (16%) of these patients had diabetes [53]. Niacin significantly reduced the risk of nonfatal MI and stroke in the Coronary Drug Project, in which 40% of the patients had evidence of abnormal glucose tolerance [54]. Lovastatin, in combination with extended release niacin, is the first fixed-dose combination product that, in dosages of up to 40 mg of niacin plus 2000 mg of niaspan, reportedly lowered LDL cholesterol and triglyceride by 47% and 41%, respectively, and increased HDL cholesterol by 30% [55].

In patients who have diabetic lipemia or severe hypertriglyceridemia, fibrates are the drug of choice; in addition, dietary and lifestyle measures should include a very low fat diet, alcohol restriction, physical activity, glycemic control, and weight management. Many patients are unable to lower triglyceride levels to a safe range (<500 mg/dL) and require the addition of niacin or fish oils. Usually, the latter is required in large dosages (to provide 3 to 6 g or more of omega-3 fatty acids) [56].

Table 5
Major on-going lipid trials with cardiovascular end points

| Study | N | Active drugs | Comments |
|-------|---|--------------|----------|
| TNT | ~10,000 | Atorvastatin, 10 or 80 mg | LDL goal: 100 versus 75 mg/dL |
| SEARCH | ~12,000 | Simvastatin, 20 or 80 mg ± B$_{12}$ and folate | LDL ± homocysteine reduction |
| IDEAL | 8888 | Simvastatin 20–40 or Atorvastatin 80 mg | Moderate versus high dose statin |
| FIELD | ~6000 | Fenofibrate or placebo | Fibrate therapy in diabetes |
| ACCORD | ~5800 | Simvastatin 20 mg ± fenofibrate | Monotherapy versus combination therapy in diabetes |

*Abbreviations:* ACCORD, Action to Control Cardiovascular Risk in Diabetes; FIELD, Fenofibrate in Lipids and Diabetes; IDEAL, The Incremental Decrease in Endpoints Through Aggressive Lipid Lowering Trial; SEARCH, Study of Effectiveness of Additional Reductions in Cholesterol and Homocysteine; TNT, Treat to New Targets.

The addition of a thiazolidinedione (TZD) is a valid approach to increasing HDL cholesterol in patients who have diabetes that requires glycemic control. Both of the available TZDs, rosiglitazone and pioglitazone, increase HDL cholesterol by 10% to 15%, based on baseline HDL levels [57]. Pioglitazone was shown to lower triglycerides but both agents are effective in correcting the LDL compositional abnormalities that are associated with insulin resistance. The results of on-going long-term trials to assess CHD outcome measures are awaited.

## References

[1] Executive Summary of The Third Report of The National Cholesterol Education Program (NCEP) Expert Panel on Detection, Evaluation, And Treatment of High Blood Cholesterol In Adults (Adult Treatment Panel III). JAMA 2001;285(19):2486–97.

[2] Haffner SM, Lehto S, Ronnemaa T, Pyorala K, Laakso M. Mortality from coronary heart disease in subjects with type 2 diabetes and in nondiabetic subjects with and without prior myocardial infarction. N Engl J Med 1998;339(4):229–34.

[3] Malmberg K, Yusuf S, Gerstein HC, Brown J, Zhao F, Hunt D, et al. Impact of diabetes on long-term prognosis in patients with unstable angina and non-Q-wave myocardial infarction: results of the OASIS (Organization to Assess Strategies for Ischemic Syndromes) Registry. Circulation 2000;102(9): 1014–9.

[4] Hu FB, Stampfer MJ, Haffner SM, Solomon CG, Willett WC, Manson JE. Elevated risk of cardiovascular disease prior to clinical diagnosis of type 2 diabetes. Diabetes Care 2002;25(7):1129–34.

[5] Stamler J, Vaccaro O, Neaton JD, Wentworth D. Diabetes, other risk factors, and 12-yr cardiovascular mortality for men screened in the Multiple Risk Factor Intervention Trial. Diabetes Care 1993; 16(2):434–44.

[6] Goldberg IJ. Clinical review 124: diabetic dyslipidemia: causes and consequences. J Clin Endocrinol Metab 2001;86(3):965–71.

[7] Taskinen MR. Diabetic dyslipidaemia: from basic research to clinical practice. Diabetologia 2003; 46(6):733–49.

[8] Garvey WT, Kwon S, Zheng D, Shaughnessy S, Wallace P, Hutto A, et al. Effects of insulin resistance and type 2 diabetes on lipoprotein subclass particle size and concentration determined by nuclear magnetic resonance. Diabetes 2003;52(2):453–62.

[9] Sniderman AD, Lamarche B, Tilley J, Seccombe D, Frohlich J. Hypertriglyceridemic hyperapoB in type 2 diabetes. Diabetes Care 2002;25(3):579–82.

[10] Wagner AM, Perez A, Zapico E, Ordonez-Llanos J. Non-HDL cholesterol and apolipoprotein B in the dyslipidemic classification of type 2 diabetic patients. Diabetes Care 2003;26(7):2048–51.

[11] Sniderman AD. Non-HDL cholesterol versus apolipoprotein B in diabetic dyslipoproteinemia: alternatives and surrogates versus the real thing. Diabetes Care 2003;26(7):2207–8.

[12] Lu W, Resnick HE, Jablonski KA, Jones KL, Jain AK, Howard WJ, et al. Non-HDL cholesterol as a predictor of cardiovascular disease in type 2 diabetes: the strong heart study. Diabetes Care 2003;26(1):16–23.

[13] Bos G, Dekker JM, Nijpels G, de Vegt F, Diamant M, Stehouwer CD, et al. A combination of high concentrations of serum triglyceride and non-high-density-lipoprotein-cholesterol is a risk factor for cardiovascular disease in subjects with abnormal glucose metabolism—The Hoorn Study. Diabetologia 2003;46(7):910–6.

[14] Schaefer EJ, Audelin MC, McNamara JR, Shah PK, Tayler T, Daly JA, et al. Comparison of fasting and postprandial plasma lipoproteins in subjects with and without coronary heart disease. Am J Cardiol 2001;88(10):1129–33.

[15] Randomised trial of cholesterol lowering in 4444 patients with coronary heart disease: the Scandinavian Simvastatin Survival Study (4S). Lancet 1994; 344(8934):1383–9.

[16] Pyorala K, Pedersen TR, Kjekshus J, Faergeman O, Olsson AG, Thorgeirsson G. Cholesterol lowering with simvastatin improves prognosis of diabetic patients with coronary heart disease. A subgroup analysis of the Scandinavian Simvastatin Survival Study (4S). Diabetes Care 1997;20(4):614–20.

[17] Haffner SM, Alexander CM, Cook TJ, Boccuzzi SJ, Musliner TA, Pedersen TR, et al. Reduced coronary events in simvastatin-treated patients with coronary heart disease and diabetes or impaired fasting glucose levels: subgroup analyses in the Scandinavian Simvastatin Survival Study. Arch Intern Med 1999;159(22):2661–7.

[18] Sacks FM, Pfeffer MA, Moye LA, Rouleau JL, Rutherford JD, Cole TG, et al. The effect of pravastatin on coronary events after myocardial infarction in patients with average cholesterol levels. Cholesterol and Recurrent Events Trial investigators. N Engl J Med 1996;335(14):1001–9.

[19] Goldberg RB, Mellies MJ, Sacks FM, Moye LA, Howard BV, Howard WJ, et al. Cardiovascular events and their reduction with pravastatin in diabetic and glucose-intolerant myocardial infarction survivors with average cholesterol levels: subgroup analyses in the cholesterol and recurrent events (CARE) trial. The Care Investigators. Circulation 1998;98(23):2513–9.

[20] Prevention of cardiovascular events and death with pravastatin in patients with coronary heart disease and a broad range of initial cholesterol levels. The Long-Term Intervention with Pravastatin in Ischaemic Disease (LIPID) Study Group. N Engl J Med 1998;339(19):1349–57.

[21] Downs JR, Clearfield M, Weis S, Whitney E, Shapiro DR, Beere PA, et al. Primary prevention of acute coronary events with lovastatin in men and women with average cholesterol levels: results of AFCAPS/TexCAPS. Air Force/Texas Coronary Atherosclerosis Prevention Study. JAMA 1998; 279(20):1615–22.

[22] MRC/BHF Heart Protection Study of cholesterol lowering with simvastatin in 20,536 high risk individuals: a randomized placebo-controlled trial. Lancet 2002;360(9326):7–22.

[23] Collins R, Armitage J, Parish S, Sleigh P, Peto R. MRC/BHF Heart Protection Study of cholesterol-lowering with simvastatin in 5963 people with diabetes: a randomised placebo-controlled trial. Lancet 2003;361(9374):2005–16.

[24] Shepherd J, Blauw GJ, Murphy MB, Bollen EL, Buckley BM, Cobbe SM, et al. Pravastatin in elderly individuals at risk of vascular disease (PROSPER): a randomised controlled trial. Lancet 2002; 360(9346):1623–30.

[25] Athyros VG, Papageorgiou AA, Mercouris BR, Anthyrou VV, Symeonidis AN, Basayannis EO, et al. Treatment with atorvastatin to the National Cholesterol Educational Program goal versus 'usual' care in secondary coronary heart disease prvention. The Greek Atorvastatin and Coronary-heart-disease Evaluation (GREACE) study. Curr Med Res Opin 2002;18(4):220–8.

[26] Sever PS, Dahlof B, Poulter NR, Wedel H, Beevers G, Caulfield M, et al. Prevention of coronary and stroke events with atorvastatin in hypertensive patients who have average or lower-than-average cholesterol concentrations, in the Anglo-Scandinavian Cardiac Outcomes Trial–Lipid Lowering Arm (ASCOT-LLA): a multicentre randomised controlled trial. Lancet 2003;361(9364):1149–58.

[27] ALLHAT Officers and Coordinators for the ALLHAT Collaborative Research Group. The Antihypertensive and Lipid-Lowering Treatment to Prevent Heart Attack Trial. Major outcomes in moderately hypercholesterolemic, hypertensive patients randomized to pravastatin vs usual care: the Antihypertensive and Lipid-Lowering Treatment to Prevent Heart Attack Trial (ALLHAT-LLT). JAMA 2002;288(23):2998–3007.

[28] Colhoun HM, Betteridge DJ, Durrington PN, et al. Primary prevention of cardiovascular disease with atorvastatin in type 2 diabetes in the Collaborative Atorvastatin Diabetes Study (CARDS): multicentre randomised placebo-controlled trial. Lancet 2004; 364(9435):685–96.

[29] Cannon CP, Braunwald E, McCabe CH, et al. Intensive versus moderate lipid lowering with statins after acute coronary syndromes. N Engl J Med 2004; 350(15):1495–504.

[30] de Lemos JA, Blazing MA, Wiviott SD, et al. Early intensive versus a delayed conservative simvastatin strategy in patients with acute coronary syndromes: phase Z of the A to Z trial. JAMA 2004;292(11): 1307–16.

[31] Hoogwerf BJ, Waness A, Cressman M, Canner J, Campeau L, Domanski M, et al. Effects of aggressive cholesterol lowering and low-dose anticoagulation on clinical and angiographic outcomes in patients with diabetes: the Post Coronary Artery Bypass Graft Trial. Diabetes 1999;48(6):1289–94.

[32] Law MR, Wald NJ, Rudnicka AR. Quantifying effect of statins on low density lipoprotein cholesterol, ischaemic heart disease, and stroke: systematic review and meta-analysis. BMJ 2003;326(7404):1423.

[33] Austin MA, Hokanson JE, Edwards KL. Hypertriglyceridemia as a cardiovascular risk factor. Am J Cardiol 1998;81(4A):7B–12B.

[34] Ballantyne CM, Olsson AG, Cook TJ, Mercuri MF, Pedersen TR, Kjekshus J. Influence of low high-density lipoprotein cholesterol and elevated triglyceride on coronary heart disease events and response to simvastatin therapy in 4S. Circulation 2001; 104(25):3046–51.

[35] Koskinen P, Manttari M, Manninen V, Huttunen JK, Heinonen OP, Frick MH. Coronary heart disease incidence in NIDDM patients in the Helsinki Heart Study. Diabetes Care 1992;15(7):820–5.

[36] Elkeles RS, Diamond JR, Poulter C, Dhanjil S, Nicolaides AN, Mahmood S, et al. Cardiovascular outcomes in type 2 diabetes. A double-blind placebo-controlled study of bezafibrate: the St. Mary's, Ealing, Northwick Park Diabetes Cardiovascular Disease Prevention (SENDCAP) Study. Diabetes Care 1998;21(4):641–8.

[37] Effect of fenofibrate on progression of coronary-artery disease in type 2 diabetes: the Diabetes Atherosclerosis Intervention Study, a randomized study. Lancet 2001;357(9260):905–10.

[38] Rubins HB, Robins SJ, Collins D, Fye CL, Anderson JW, Elam MB, et al. Gemfibrozil for the secondary prevention of coronary heart disease in men with low levels of high-density lipoprotein cholesterol. Veterans Affairs High-Density Lipoprotein Cholesterol Intervention Trial Study Group. N Engl J Med 1999;341(6):410–8.

[39] Rubins HB, Robins SJ, Collins D, Nelson DB, Elam MB, Schaefer EJ, et al. Diabetes, plasma insulin, and cardiovascular disease: subgroup analysis from the Department of Veterans Affairs high-density lipoprotein intervention trial (VA-HIT). Arch Intern Med 2002;162(22):2597–604.

[40] Robins SJ, Rubins HB, Faas FH, Schaefer EJ, Elam MB, Anderson JW, et al. Insulin resistance and cardiovascular events with low HDL cholesterol: the Veterans Affairs HDL Intervention Trial (VA-HIT). Diabetes Care 2003;26(5):1513–7.

[41] Robins SJ, Collins D, Wittes JT, Papademetriou V, Deedwania PC, Schaefer EJ, et al. Relation of gemfibrozil treatment and lipid levels with major coronary events: VA-HIT: a randomized controlled trial. JAMA 2001;285(12):1585–91.

[42] Haffner SM. Management of dyslipidemia in adults with diabetes. Diabetes Care 2003;26(Suppl 1): S83–6.

[43] Grundy SM, Cleeman JI, Merz CN, et al. Implications of recent clinical trials for the National Cholesterol Education Program Adult Treatment Panel III guidelines. Circulation 2004;110(2):227–39.

[44] Jenkins DJ, Kendall CW, Marchie A, Faulkner DA, Wong JM, de Souza R, et al. Effects of a dietary portfolio of cholesterol-lowering foods vs lovastatin on serum lipids and C-reactive protein. JAMA 2003; 290(4):502–10.

[45] Jones PH, Davidson MH, Stein EA, Bays HE, McKenney JM, Miller E, et al. Comparison of the efficacy and safety of rosuvastatin versus atorvastatin, simvastatin, and pravastatin across doses (STELLAR* Trial). Am J Cardiol 2003;92(2): 152–60.

[46] Kreisberg RA, Oberman A. Medical management of hyperlipidemia/dyslipidemia. J Clin Endocrinol Metab 2003;88(6):2445–61.

[47] Marcus A. Current lipid-lowering strategies for the treatment of diabetic dyslipidemia: an integrated approach to therapy. Endocrinologist 2001;11:368–83.

[48] Elam MB, Hunninghake DB, Davis KB, Garg R, Johnson C, Egan D, et al. Effect of niacin on lipid and lipoprotein levels and glycemic control in patients with diabetes and peripheral arterial disease: the ADMIT study: a randomized trial. Arterial Disease Multiple Intervention Trial. JAMA 2000; 284(10):1263–70.

[49] Grundy SM, Vega GL, McGovern ME, Tulloch BR, Kendall DM, Fitz-Patrick D, et al. Efficacy, safety, and tolerability of once-daily niacin for the treatment of dyslipidemia associated with type 2 diabetes: results of the assessment of diabetes control and evaluation of the efficacy of niaspan trial. Arch Intern Med 2002;162(14):1568–76.

[50] Gagne C, Bays HE, Weiss SR, Mata P, Quinto K, Melino M, et al. Efficacy and safety of ezetimibe added to ongoing statin therapy for treatment of patients with primary hypercholesterolemia. Am J Cardiol 2002;90(10):1084–91.

[51] Athyros VG, Papageorgiou AA, Athyrou VV, Demitriadis DS, Kontopoulos AG. Atorvastatin and micronized fenofibrate alone and in combination in type 2 diabetes with combined hyperlipidemia. Diabetes Care 2002;25(7):1198–202.

[52] Neil A, Wheeler F, Cull C, Manley S, Keenan J, Holman R. Combination statin and fibrate therapy in type 2 diabetes: results from the Lipids in Diabetes Study. Diabetes 2003;52(Suppl 1):A74.

[53] Brown BG, Zhao XQ, Chait A, Fisher LD, Cheung MC, Morse JS, et al. Simvastatin and niacin, antioxidant vitamins, or the combination for the prevention of coronary disease. N Engl J Med 2001; 345(22):1583–92.

[54] Canner PL, Furberg CD, McGovern ME. Niacin decreases myocardial infarction and total mortality in patients with impaired fasting glucose or glucose i tolerance: results from the Coronary Drug Project. Circulation 2002;106(suppl 2) II–636.

[55] Kashyap ML, McGovern ME, Berra K, Guyton JR, Kwiterovich PO, Harper WL, et al. Long-term safety and efficacy of a once-daily niacin/lovastatin formulation for patients with dyslipidemia. Am J Cardiol 2002;89(6):672–8.

[56] Kris-Etherton PM, Harris WS, Appel LJ. Fish consumption, fish oil, omega-3 fatty acids, and cardiovascular disease. Arterioscler Thromb Vasc Biol 2003;23(2):20–30.

[57] Khan MA, St Peter JV, Xue JL. A prospective, randomized comparison of the metabolic effects of pioglitazone or rosiglitazone in patients with type 2 diabetes who were previously treated with troglitazone. Diabetes Care 2002;25(4):708–11.

ELSEVIER
SAUNDERS

Cardiol Clin 23 (2005) 165–183

CARDIOLOGY
CLINICS

# The Renin Angiotensin System as a Therapeutic Target to Prevent Diabetes and its Complications

Kris Vijayaraghavan, MD[a,b,c],
Prakash C. Deedwania, MD, FACC, FACP, FCCP, FAHA[d,*]

[a]Research and Heart Failure Program, Scottsdale Cardiovascular Research Institute,
Scottsdale, AZ 85251, USA
[b]Congestive Heart Failure Clinic, Arizona Heart Hospital, 1930 Thomas Road, Phoenix, AZ 85006, USA
[c]Midwestern Osteopathic School of Medicine, 19555 North 59th Avenue, Glendale, AZ 85308, USA
[d]Department of Medicine, VA Central California Health Care System/University Medical Center,
University of California, San Francisco Program at Fresno, 2615 East Clinton Avenue, Fresno, CA 93703, USA

### The burden of diabetes

Type 2 diabetes is a complex chronic disease with increasing microvascular and macrovascular complications imposing a significant public health and economic burden [1]. Even though a number of efficacious treatments are available, suboptimal applications of these in clinical practice has led to gaps in diabetes prevention and management. Barriers for providers include time constraints, forgetfulness, a perception of patients as noncompliant, and inadequate knowledge of outcomes from clinical trials. Barriers for patients include inadequate comprehension of the gravity of the disease, little motivation toward prevention of diabetes and its complications, insufficient time, and lack of socioeconomic resources and support [2–4]. The prevalence of diabetes has increased by 61% from 1990 to 2001 with type 2 diabetes accounting for 95% of this increase [5]. The annual cost of the disease is estimated at $132 billion accounting for more than 10% of the United States health care expenditure. Moreover, the lifetime risk for developing diabetes among Americans born in year 2000 is 32.8% for men and 38.5% for women [6]. Hence, there is an urgent need to prevent the

* Corresponding author. VACCHCS/UCSF, 2615 East Clinton Avenue, Fresno, CA 93703.
E-mail address: deed@ucsfresno.edu (P.C. Deedwania).

onset of diabetes in the high-risk population. This review addresses the evidence of prevention through lifestyle modification, its challenges, and additional means through pharmacologic interventions specifically targeting the renin angiotensin aldosterone system (RAAS) that may reduce the overall public and economic health burden.

### Risk factors for diabetes

The increase in prevalence of type 2 diabetes is paralleled by the rising rate of obesity and metabolic syndrome. As body mass index (BMI) increases, the risk of developing type 2 diabetes increases correspondingly. The prevalence of type 2 diabetes is three to seven times higher in obese patients and is 20 times higher in those with a BMI greater 35 kg/m$^2$ than in those with a BMI between 18.5 and 24.9 kg/m$^2$ [7–8]. This increased prevalence, however, may vary among ethnic groups. Obesity is a component of metabolic syndrome. The National Cholesterol Education Program Adult Treatment Panel (NECP-ATP III) defines metabolic syndrome using the objective clinical criteria given in Table 1 [9].

Metabolic syndrome is defined as the presence of any three of the risk factors. The clustering of risk factors associated with this syndrome predicts development of manifest diabetes and cardiovascular disease. Hence, prevention of type 2 diabetes should aim to treat and prevent components of

Table 1
Clinical criteria for metabolic syndrome

| Risk factor | Definition |
| --- | --- |
| Abdominal obesity | Men: waist circumference > 40 in |
| | Women: waist circumference > 35 in |
| Elevated triglycerides | ≥ 150 mg/dL |
| HDL cholesterol | Men: < 40 mg/dL |
| | Women: < 50 mg/dL |
| Elevated blood pressure | ≥ 130 mm Hg systolic and/or ≥ 85 mm Hg diastolic or use of antihypertensive agent |
| Fasting blood sugar | ≥ 110 mg/dL or use of hypoglycemic agent |

metabolic syndrome. Other risk factors for type 2 diabetes mellitus include age of 45 years or older, family history of diabetes (parent or siblings), physical inactivity, ethnicity (eg, Afro-American, Hispanic, Native American, Asian American, or Pacific Islander), impaired glucose tolerance, history of gestational diabetes or delivery of a baby weighing more than 9 lbs, hypertension (blood pressure ≥ 140/90 mm Hg in adults), high-density lipoprotein (HDL) cholesterol level below 35 mg/dL and triglyceride level above 250 mg/dL, polycystic ovary syndrome, and history of vascular disease [10]. Park and Edington [11] applied a prediction model using sequential multilayered perception neural network architecture. High BMI was the most significant risk factor; other significant factors that predicted risk over time with variations in trajectory were elevated blood pressure, stress, elevated cholesterol levels, and fatty food intake.

## Lifestyle modifications and its effects on prevention

Multiple clinical trials have tested lifestyle modification to prevent type 2 diabetes. The inclusion criteria for all trials were impaired glucose tolerance based on two blood glucose measurements: a fasting value of less than 126 mg/dL, and a glucose value of 140 to 200 mg/dL 2 hours after consumption of 75 g of glucose. In the United Kingdom, Jarrett et al in the Borderline Diabetes Study and Keen et al in the Bedford Survey found no effect of dietary modification on preventing diabetes [12]. A Swedish study, however, found that diabetes counseling and tolbutamide reduced the incidence of diabetes, although intention-to-treat

analysis was not performed [13]. More recently, the three studies of primary prevention that used lifestyle intervention have shown significant results. The Finnish Diabetes Prevention Study, the Da Qing Imaired Glucose Tolerance and Diabetes Study, and the Diabetes Prevention Program revealed that aggressive dietary intervention and an exercise program reduced the incidence of diabetes by 58%, 42%, and 58%, respectively, compared with controls [14–16]. The details are shown in Table 2.

Implementing lifestyle intervention at an individual level, especially in obese persons and those at high risk, is challenging. It is accompanied by deficiencies, primarily in motivation, both at the physician and patient level. Changes in health behavior have always been associated with efforts that are ephemeral, leading to a rebound increase in body weight. This increase, in turn, leads to loss of benefits that may have been accrued [17–18]. In addition, patients and providers encounter barriers in the health care system that make it difficult to translate results from the research setting into clinical practice. Many studies have assessed delivery of multifaceted, system-oriented, and integrated approaches aimed at primary prevention of type 2 diabetes [17–19]. Unfortunately, the long-term success of these programs has been disenchanting. Reductions in cardiovascular risk were suboptimal, without any overall reduction in mortality [20,21].

In addition, lifestyle changes are expensive. The most recent analysis from the Diabetes Prevention Program showed that in clinical practice the cost per case of diabetes delayed or prevented was similar for metformin ($14,300) and lifestyle interventions ($13,200) [22]. Hence it is important to consider all means available, including pharmacologic interventions, to prevent the development of diabetes. Prevention of diabetes by use of metformin, acarbose, and thiazolidinediones has been described elsewhere. This article focuses on RAAS inhibition as a therapeutic model to prevent diabetes.

## The renin angiotensin aldosterone system as a therapeutic target

Angiotensin-converting enzyme (ACE) inhibitors were initially developed in the late 1970s for treatment of hypertension. Their use has since been expanded to heart failure, postmyocardial infarction, and renal disease. ACE inhibitors, by

Table 2
Studies on prevention of type 2 diabetes with life style modifications

| Variables | Finnish Diabetes Prevention Study [15] | Da Qing Impaired Glucose Tolerance and Diabetes Study [14] | Diabetes Prevention Program [16] |
|---|---|---|---|
| N | 522 | 520 | 3234 |
| Mean age $\pm$ 1 SD | 55 $\pm$ 7 | 45 $\pm$ 9.1 | 50.6 $\pm$ 10.7 |
| Women (%) | 67 | 47 | 68 |
| Mean BMI kg/m$^2$ | 31.2 $\pm$ 4.6 | 25.8 $\pm$ 3.8 | 34 $\pm$ 6.7 |
| Study duration (yrs) | 3.2 | 6 | 2.8 |
| White (%) | – | – | 55 |
| Other ethnic groups (%) | – | – | 45 |
| Study groups | control intervention (weight loss, diet, physical activity) | control diet exercise diet + exercise | placebo metformin life style intervention (weight loss, diet, physical activity) |
| Adjusted reduction in incidence of type 2 diabetes (%) | 58 | diet 31 exercise 46 diet + exercise 42 | metformin 31 life style intervention 58 |

blocking the conversion of angiotensin I to angiotensin II and by catalyzing the breakdown of bradykinin, exert numerous beneficial effects that maintain blood pressure and salt and water homeostasis. In addition, the vasodilating, anti-inflammatory, plaque-stabilizing, antithrombotic, and antiproliferative properties of ACE inhibitors produce salutary effects. Numerous studies have demonstrated a significant benefit with use of ACE inhibition. The Cooperative North Scandinavian Enalapril Survival Study (CONSENSUS), the Studies on Left Ventricular Dysfunction (SOLVD) treatment and prevention study, and the Vasodilator-Heart Failure Trial II (V-HeFT II) demonstrated significant overall mortality reduction in patients with congestive heart failure treated with enalapril. The Survival and Ventricular Enlargement trial (SAVE) and the International Study of Infarct Survival 4 (ISIS-4) study also revealed a survival benefit in postmyocardial infarction patients treated with captopril. In the Acute Infarction Ramipril Efficacy (AIRE) study, mortality was reduced in patients with recent myocardial infarction and overt congestive heart failure who were treated with ramipril. In addition, ramipril provided significant benefit in cardiovascular outcomes and mortality in patients with cardiovascular disease or diabetes and one other risk factor in the AIRE study. Lisinopril, trandolapril, and zofenopril improved survival in patients with acute myocardial infarction, recent myocardial infarction with left ventricular dysfunction, and acute myocardial infarction, respectively (Table 3) [23–32]. Angiotensin receptor

blockers also have shown significant benefit in both cardiovascular and renal outcomes (Table 4) [33–45]. Losartan compared with atenolol in patients with hypertension and left ventricular hypertrophy showed reduction in composite cardiovascular mortality, myocardial infarction, and stroke in the Losartan Intervention for Endpoint (LIFE) study (relative risk [RR], 13%; $P = 0.021$) [33]; in the Optimal Trial in Myocardial Infarction with Angiotensin II Antagonist Losartan (OPTIMAAL) study, but losartan showed no difference in all-cause mortality compared with captopril in in subjects with acute myocardial infarction [38]. Also, no difference in mortality was noted with losartan compared with captoril in the ELITE II Losartan Heart Failure Survival Study of congestive heart failure [40]. The Reduction of End Points in Non-Insulin-Dependent Diabetes Mellitus with the Angiotensin II Antagonist Losartan (RENAAL) study found a significant reduction of serum creatinine levels, end-stage renal disease, and death with losartan compared with placebo in patients with diabetic nephropathy (RR, 16%; $P = 0.02$) [37]. The Valsartan Heart Failure Trial (Val HeFT) compared valsartan with placebo for treatment of heart failure and revealed no difference in mortality but found a significant reduction in hospitalization [41]. When valsartan was added to captopril following acute myocardial infarction in the Valsartan in Acute Myocardial Infarction Trial (VALIANT) study, there was no difference in mortality or composite endpoints compared with either of the medications alone [39]. The Valsartan Antihypertensive Long-term use

Table 3
Summary of angiotensin-converting enzyme inhibitor clinical trials

| Trial | ACE inhibitor | Patient group | Outcome |
|---|---|---|---|
| CONSENSUS (N = 253) | enalapril versus placebo | NYHA IV, CHF | ↓ overall mortality |
| SOLVD, treatment arm (N = 2569) | enalapril versus placebo | NYHA II & III, CHF | ↓ overall mortality |
| V-HeFT II (N = 804) | enalapril versus hydralazine isosorbide | NYHA II & III, CHF | ↓ overall mortality |
| SAVE (N = 2231) | captopril versus placebo | recent MI with asymptomatic LVD | ↓ overall mortality |
| SOLVD, prevention arm (N = 4228) | enalapril versus placebo | asymptomatic LVD | ↓ death and hospitalization from CHF |
| AIRE (N = 2006) | ramipril versus placebo | recent MI with overt CHF | ↓ overall mortality |
| ISIS-4 (N > 50,000) | captopril versus placebo | acute MI | ↓ overall mortality |
| GISSI-3 (N = 19,394) | lisinopril versus open control | acute MI | ↓ overall mortality |
| TRACE (N = 1749) | trandolapril versus placebo | recent MI with LVD | ↓ overall mortality |
| SMILE (N = 1556) | zofenopril versus placebo | acute MI | ↓ overall mortality |

*Definitions:* CHF, congestive heart failure; GISSI-3, Gruppo Italiano per lo Studio della Sopravvivvenza nell'Infarto Miocardica III; LVD, left ventricular dysfunction; MI, myocardial infarction; NYHA, New York Heart Association; SMILE, Survival of Myocardial Infarction Long-Term Evaluation trial; TRACE, Trandolapril Cardiac Evaluation trial.
*From* Refs. [23–32].

Evaluation (VALUE) trial found no difference in composite endpoints of mortality and morbidity between valsartan and amlodipine [34]. Irbesartan was compared with amlodipine (in the IDNT study) [35] and with placebo (in the Irbesartan MicroAlbuminuria [IRMA] study) [36] in patients with diabetic nephropathy. [36], Irbesartan showed significant reduction of overt proteinuria, end-stage renal disease and doubling of serum creatinine. In the Candesartan in Heart Failure Assessment of Reduction in Mortality and Morbidity (CHARM) study, candesartan also showed reduction in composite endpoints of mortality and morbidity compared with placebo in heart failure patients with left ventricular dysfunction (Table 4) [42–45].

The rationale for considering RAAS inhibition in patients at risk of developing diabetes is based on the following concepts:

1. The role of activation of RAAS, the ensuing detrimental effects on cardiovascular and renal disease, and extensive evidence indicating that ACE inhibition favorably affects the heart, vasculature, and kidney, with improved patient outcomes
2. The deleterious effects of angiotensin II on vasculature and its role in endothelial dysfunction
3. The close relationship between insulin resistance (a precursor of diabetes and cardiovascular disease) and endothelial dysfunction

4. The pathways of insulin signaling and angiotensin II in the vascular wall and the intracellular crosstalk between these signaling pathways that lends theoretical credence to the concept of diabetes prevention through RAAS blockade
5. Clinical evidence in secondary outcomes of prevention of new onset of diabetes from studies on RAAS inhibition
6. Clinical studies of ACE/angiotensin receptor blocker (ARB) inhibition and outcomes of markers of insulin resistance

## Role of renin angiotensin aldosterone system activation

Angiotensin II is formed from the substrate angiotensinogen through a series of steps. Renin catalyzes the conversion of angiotensinogen to angiotensin I, which is subsequently hydrolyzed by ACE to form angiotensin II. Alternate pathways, such as tissue plasminogen activator, cathepsin G, and tonin, also convert angiotensinogen directly to angiotensin II, whereas angiotensin I is also catalyzed to angiotensin II by chymase and cathepsin G [46,47]. Angiotensin II mediates deleterious effects by binding specific receptors located on the cell membrane. Angiotensin II receptor type I mediates the biologic activities that are harmful to the tissues. The expression of angiotensin II receptor type II is

Table 4
Angiotensin receptor blockers in clinical trials

| Condition | Trial | Drugs | N | Duration | Outcome | Result |
|---|---|---|---|---|---|---|
| LVH and hypertension | LIFE [33] | losartan, 50–100 mg, versus atenolol, 50–100 mg | 9193 | 5 yr | composite CV mortality, MI, stroke | 13% RR ($P = 0.021$) |
| hypertension | VALUE [34] | valsartan, up to 160 mg, versus amlodipine, up to 10 mg | 15,245 | 4.2 yr | composite endpoint of mortality and morbidity | no difference between valsartan and amlodipine |
| diabetic nephropathy | IDNT [35] | irbesartan, up to 300 mg, versus amlodipine, up to 10 mg, versus placebo | 1715 | 2.6 yr | doubling of SCR, ESRD or death | 20% lower than placebo ($P = 0.02$) 23% lower than amlodipine ($P = 0.006$) |
| diabetic nephropathy | IRMA [36] | irbesartan, 150 mg or 300 mg, versus placebo | 590 | 3 mo | albuminuria, overt proteinuria | 24% lower albumin excretion with 150 mg irbesartan ($P < 0.001$), 38% lower albumin excretion with 300 mg irbasartan ($P < 0.001$), 70% reduction of overt proteinuria ($P < 0.001$) |
| diabetic nephropathy | RENAAL [37] | Losartan, 50–100 mg, versus placebo | 1513 | 3.4 yr | doubling of SCR, ESRD or death | 16% reduction of composite ($P = 0.02$), 25% reduction in doubling of SCR, 28% reduction in ESRD, no change in deaths |
| acute MI | OPTIMAAL [38] | Losartan, 50 mg/d, or captopril, 50 mg tid | 5477 | 6 mo | all-cause mortality, SCD and total and NFMI | no difference between captopril and losartan, 13.3% death with captopril versus 15.3% death with losartan ($P = 0.03$) |
| acute MI | VALIANT [39] | Valsartan, 160 mg bid, captopril 50 mg tid, or combinations of valsartan, 80mg bid, and captopril, 50 mg tid | 14,703 | 2.1 yr | all-cause mortality, CV death, MI, hospitalization to CHF | no difference between groups |
| CHF | ELITE II [40] | losartan 50 mg/d, captopril, 50 mg tid | 3152 | 555 d | all-cause mortality | no difference |
| CHF | ValHeft [41] | valsartan 160 mg, placebo | 5010 | | mortality and composite endpoint of mortality and morbidity | no difference in mortality, improvement in hospitalization with valsartan |
| CHF | CHARM, overall [42] | cansesartan 32 mg/d, placebo | 7601 | 2 yr | all-cause mortality | 17% reduction, statistically significant |
| CHF | CHARM, alternate [43] | cansesartan 32 mg/d, placebo | 2028 | 33.7 mo | composite of CV death at hospital | 23% reduction, statistically significant |
| CHF | CHARM, added [44] | cansesartan 32 mg/d, placebo | 2548 | 41 mo | composite | 15% reduction, statistically significant |
| CHF | CHARM, preserved [45] | cansesartan 32 mg/d, placebo | 3023 | 36.6 mo | CV death or hospitalization | 11% reduction, statistically significant |

*Definitions:* CHF, congestive heart failure; CV, cardiovascular; LVH, left ventricular hypertension; IDNT, Irbesartan Diabetic Nephropathy Trial; MI, myocardial infarction.

less well studied but seems to mediate beneficial effects that include vasodilation, inhibition of cell growth, and proliferation as well as cell differentiation [48,49]. The differential effects are shown in Fig. 1. The sequential progression of cardiovascular disease begins with the risk factors of hypertension, diabetes, smoking, metabolic syndrome, and dyslipidemia. These risk factors are independently associated with levels of angiotensin II that in turn trigger the cascade of events. Progression to atherosclerotic disease and left ventricular hypertrophy leads to plaque destabilization in the face of uncontrolled risk factors, with acute coronary syndrome and myocardial infarction as the sequelae [50]. Loss of cardiac muscle eventually leads to remodeling of the left ventricle progressing relentlessly to heart failure and end-stage cardiomyopathy (Fig. 2).

## Role of the renin angiotensin aldosterone system in vascular endothelial function

The endothelium has numerous vital functions. First, it acts as a permeability barrier preventing exocytosis of macrophage and small, dense low-density lipoprotein (LDL) entering the subendothelial layer from initiating the genesis of the fatty streak, the first step in atherosclerosis. Second, it is important in maintaining vascular tone by releasing angiotensin II and endothelin, powerful vasoconstrictors, and balancing that release by the release of nitric oxide, a potent vasodilator. The endothelium also plays an active role in hemostasis, mediating coagulation by inhibiting platelet aggregation and by releasing von Willebrand's factor, tissue plasminogen activator (PAI), and RAAS. It also releases cell adhesion molecules and inflammatory cytokines such as interleukin-6, tumor necrosis factor (TNF) alpha, and others that are involved in the process of atherosclerosis. Finally, it acts as a transducer of biomechanical forces and prevents shear stress from denuding the endothelial layer to allow plaque accumulation (Fig. 3) [51,52]. Angiotensin II contributes to endothelial dysfunction by increasing oxidative stress, attenuating chemoattractants, and increasing adhesion molecule expression leading to inflammation [53]. In addition, angiotensin II can

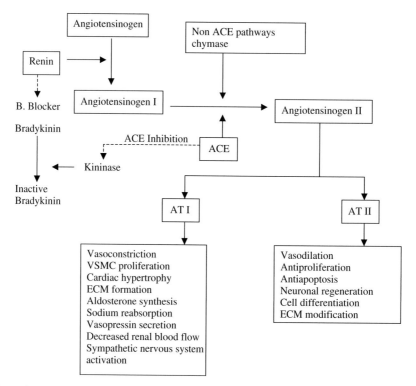

Fig. 1. Renin angiotension aldersterone system pathway. AT I, angiotensin receptor type I; AT II, angiotensin receptor type II; ECM, extracellular matrix; VSMC, vascular smooth muscle cell.

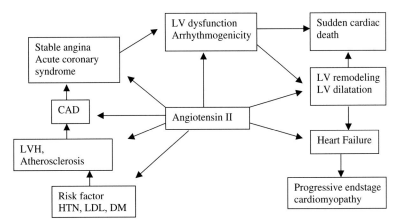

Fig. 2. Angiotensin II and the sequential progression of cardiovascular disease. CAD, coronary artery disease; DM, diabetes mellitus; HTN, hypertension; LVH, left ventricular hypertrophy.

exert proliferative and prothrombotic activity, producing superoxide radicals that scavenge nitric oxide and reducing vasodilation [54]. There is evidence that an increased expression of ACE is present in endothelial growth arrest [54]. ACE is induced by glucocorticoids in vascular smooth muscle [55]. Activation of ACE induces PAI-1 levels that contribute to atherothrombosis [56]. Bradykinin, which is unopposed with blockade of ACE, has significant beneficial effects on endothelium, primarily from its powerful vasodilating properties [57,58]. Thus, there is evidence that accumulation of angiotensin II impairs endothelial function and enhances atherogenic process.

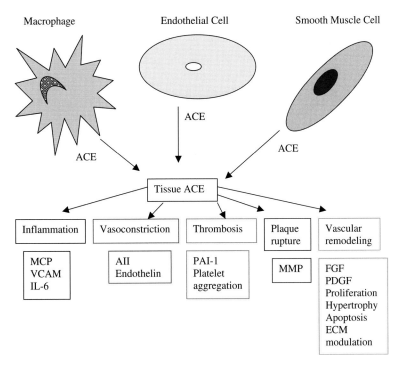

Fig. 3. Role of angiotension-converting enzyme in vascular function. AII, angiotensin II; ECM, extracellular matrix; FGF, fibroblast growth factor; MCP, monocyte chemotactic protein; MMP, matrix metalloproteinase; PDGF, platelet-derived growth factor; VCAM, vascular cell adhesion molecule.

### Interaction between angiotensin, endothelium, and insulin resistance

Insulin resistance is associated with metabolic syndrome, which increases the risk of adverse cardiovascular outcomes. There is definitive evidence that insulin resistance and endothelial dysfunction progress in parallel. As insulin resistance progresses to clinical metabolic syndrome, impaired glucose tolerance, and development of diabetes, there is a parallel track that leads from endothelial dysfunction to inflammation, with increased oxidative stress leading to overt atherosclerotic disease. Insulin resistance has been shown to interact with this parallel track of endothelial dysfunction through the accumulation of free fatty acids, proinflammatory adipokines, and TNF alpha [59]. In addition, increased oxidative stress, oxidation of LDL, the reduction of HDL, and the development of hypertension, hyperuricemia, and hyperglycemia contribute to the mechanisms of underlying endothelial dysfunction in insulin resistance [51].

Because angiotensin II plays a significant role in endothelial dysfunction, the interplay of angiotensin II in glucose homeostasis has been of significant interest to biochemical and molecular biologists. The relationships between angiotensin II and insulin signaling pathways are becoming evident in preclinical studies. Insulin binds to the cell surface receptor tyrosine kinase, which leads to autophosphorylation of the tyrosine residue that turns on the insulin signaling pathways. The initial step is activation of phosphatidyl inositol kinase (PI-3K) pathway, which is important for glucose transport in skeletal muscle. In addition, this pathway enhances nitric oxide production and insulin-induced vasodilatory response [60,61]. The second pathway that is activated is the mitogen activated protein kinase (MAPK). This pathway promotes vascular smooth muscle cell proliferation and migration induced by insulin, thrombin, and platelet derived growth factors (Fig. 4). In addition, a third pathway is triggered that leads to activation of P70 S6 kinase, a regulator of protein synthesis [62–64].

Angiotensin II plays an important role in signaling pathways for maintaining structure and function of the heart. Angiotensin I stimulation results in activation of the MAPK, PI-3K, and tyrosine phosphorylation both in vivo and vitro. In the heart, angiotensin II blocks insulin-induced PI-3K but stimulates MAPK, thus inhibiting the metabolic but not the proliferative

effects of insulin [65]. This crosstalk between the two signaling pathways may play a pivotal role in explaining how cardiovascular and neuroendocrine physiology relate to each other and thus explain the role of angiotensin II blockade in insulin resistance and prevention of diabetes.

### Improvement of endothelial function

Endothelial dysfunction leads to defects in insulin-mediated glucose uptake. Blockade of vascular nitric oxide synthesis with L-arginine analogue also impairs endothelial dependent vasodilation. Endothelial function improves with exercise, a low-fat, low-carbohydrate diet, and with use of statins and ACE inhibitors (Table 5) [29,59,67]. Angiotensin I blockade has not shown any improvement of endothelial dysfunction, but benefit has been noted with peroxisome proliferator activated receptor gamma (PPAR-$\gamma$) stimulator, antioxidants, hormone replacement therapy, and L-arginine [66,68,69]. In addition, the ACE inhibitor quinapril significantly improved endothelial function in multiple studies, both in normotensive volunteers and in subjects with coronary artery disease [70–77].

### Is lifestyle modification adequate to prevent onset of diabetes

Metabolic syndrome carries with it the underlying pathophysiologic feature of insulin resistance with tissue resistance to insulin action, compensatory hyperinsulinemia, and excessive circulating free fatty acids [78,79]. In addition, cardiovascular risk factors of low HDL and high triglyceride levels, hypertension, and lack of physical activity have all been shown to be predictors of non–insulin-dependent diabetes [80]. The relationships between metabolic syndrome and cardiovascular mortality as well as chronic complications of type 2 diabetes have been well described [81,82]. Several studies have shown impaired glucose tolerance to be a predictor of progression to type 2 diabetes [83–85]. In addition, in one study, adiponectin was an independent predictor of type 2 diabetes [86]. It follows, then, that aggressive intervention in patients with impaired glucose tolerance or metabolic syndrome would translate to diabetes prevention. In addition to the Da Qing study, the Finnish diabetes prevention study and the diabetes prevention program (DPP), several smaller studies

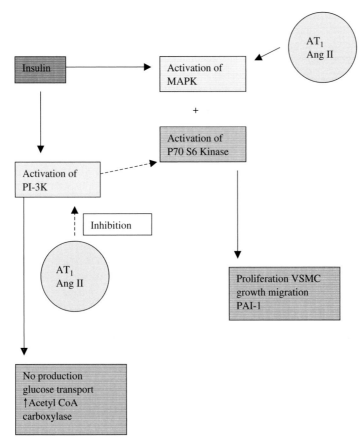

Fig. 4. Angiotensin II, insulin signaling and crosstalk. Ang I, angiotensin II; VSMC, vascular smooth muscle cell.

have reflected the benefit of lifestyle modifications [87–92]. Weight loss programs, dietary modification, and aggressive exercise regimens are fraught with challenges, however [93,94]. As urbanization becomes more widespread, exercise as a modality

for weight loss will become increasingly difficult and possibly destined to failure. A group of obese Hawaiians lost 7.8 kg in 3 weeks when they changed their diet to ad libitum feeding of their traditional diet, which provided only 7% of energy

Table 5
Endothelial function improvement and association with prevention of type 2 diabetes

| Variable | Prevention of cardiovascular disease | Improvement of endothelial function | Prevention of new-onset type 2 diabetes | Reference |
|---|---|---|---|---|
| Exercise and diet | + | + | + | [59] |
| Statins | + | + | NK | [67] |
| Ace inhibitors | + | + | + | [29] |
| AT1 blocker | + | NK | + | [33] |
| PPAR-$\gamma$ gamma stimulator | NK | + | + | [68,69] |
| Antioxidants | - | + | NK | [66] |
| HRT | - | + | NK | [66] |
| Largininine | NK | + | NK | [66] |

*Definitions:* AT1, angiotensin 1; CVD, cardiovascular disease; HRT, hormone replacement therapy; NK, not known.

as fat, [95]. This change was accomplished without increased exercise, a result that calls into question the value and need for exercise. Weight loss, however, is difficult to accomplish, and, if accomplished, to maintain, so one cannot assume that such strategies to prevent the onset of diabetes are inexpensive. Even in the DPP study, the cost per case of diabetes delayed was similar for lifestyle change and metformin. Pharmacologic interventions that might delay the onset of diabetes should not be ignored but should be considered the context of concurrent lifestyle modifications. The following evidence-based discussion sheds some light on RAAS inhibition and outcomes of new-onset diabetes.

## Clinical studies on renin angiotensin aldosterone system inhibition and outcomes of new onset diabetes

ACE inhibitors and ARBs have been studied extensively in hypertension, congestive heart failure, coronary artery disease, and renal disease (Table 6). Both drugs consistently reduce risk of coronary events (particularly ACE inhibitors), stroke, and diabetic complications of microvascular disease. In addition, secondary endpoints of some of these studies have suggested reduced incidence of new-onset diabetes. In the Heart Outcomes Prevention Evaluation (HOPE), the incidence of diabetes was 34% lower in the ramipril-treated group than in the group receiving

Table 6
Tissue angiotensin-converting enzyme inhibition and endothelial function

| Study | ACE inhibitor | Characteristics of study subject | Outcome |
|---|---|---|---|
| Saris et al [70] | enalapril | Normotensive male volunteers | inhibition of contractile effects of AI; reduction in fractional conversion of AI to AII |
| Lyons et al [71] | quinapril, enalapril | Normotensive male volunteers | quinapril, but not enalapril, significantly inhibited AII-induced vasoconstriction |
| Padmanabhan et al [72] | enalaprilat | Normotensive male volunteers | enalaprilat failed to inhibit the contractile response to AI |
| Hornig et al [73] | quinaprilat, enalaprilat | CHF patients | endothelial-dependent dilation was improved with quinaprilat, but not with enalaprilat |
| Prasad et al [74] | enalaprilat | CAD patients | enalaprilat significantly potentiated bradykinin-mediated femoral vasodilation |
| Mancini et al (TREND) [75] | quinapril | CAD patients with preserved LVF | increased coronary artery dilation; increased endothelial function in smokers and those with elevated LDL cholesterol |
| Anderson et al (BANFF) [76] | quinapril, enalapril, losartan, amlodipine | CAD patients with preserved LVF | only quinapril significantly improved endothelial function |
| Oosterga et al (QUO VADIS-1) [77] | quinapril, captopril | CAD patients with preserved LVF | quinapril, but not captopril, blocks AI conversion to AII in vascular preparations |

*Definitions:* AI, angiotensin I; AII, antiotensin II; CAD, coronary artery disease; CHF, congestive heart failure; LVF, left ventricular function.

*Adapted from* Vascular Biology Working Group website. Available at: VBWG.org. Accessed November 12, 2004.

placebo [29,96]. In the LIFE study comparing losartan with atenolol for treating hypertension with left ventricular hypertrophy, losartan was associated with a 25% reduction in new-onset diabetes compared with atenolol [33,98]. Even in the more recent Antihypertensive and Lipid-Lowering Treatment to Prevent Heart Attack Trial, the incidence of new-onset diabetes was significantly lower in the lisinopril arm than in the chlorthalidone arm [97]. The chlorthalidone arm had 302 cases of new-onset diabetes out of 9733 subjects, whereas the lisinopril arm had only 119 patients with new-onset diabetes out of 5840 participants, providing a relative risk of 0.66 (confidence interval [CI], 0.53–0.81). In the CHARM study, candesartan reduced the onset of diabetes by 19% (RR, 0.81; CI, 0.66–0.97) compared with placebo when used in patients with chronic heart failure [42]. The Antihypertensive Treatment and Lipid Profile in a North of Sweden Efficacy Evaluation (ALLHAT) study, which compared candesartan with hydrochlorothiazide, found that candesartan decreased the incidence of new-onset diabetes significantly (RR, 0.13; CI, 0.02–0.97; $P = 0.03$) [99]. The SOLVD study recently analyzed data on new-onset diabetes in the enalapril group that was compared with placebo for treatment of chronic heart failure. There was a significant reduction (RR, 0.26; CI, 0.13–0.53) of new-onset of diabetes with use of enalapril [22,23]. The results of the more recent VALUE trial indicate a 23% reduction (RR, 0.77; CI, 0.69–0.86;

$P < 0.001$) in new-onset of diabetes in hypertensive patients treated with valsartan, as compared with amlodipine [34]. The Study on Cognition and Prognosis in the Elderly by the Captopril Prevention Project (CAPP) and the Cardiovascular Events in Elderly Patients with Isolated Systolic Hypertension (STOP-HTN) study, on the other hand, showed no difference between use of ACE inhibitors or ARBs and control in new-onset of diabetes (Table 7) [100–102]. Possible mechanisms responsible for the reduced incidence of diabetes in these trials include improvement in insulin-mediated glucose uptake, enhanced endothelial function, increased nitric oxide activation, reduced inflammatory response, and increased bradykinin levels [103–106].

## Clinical studies of renin angiotensin aldosterone system inhibition and outcomes of insulin resistance

ACE inhibition with captopril improves insulin sensitivity [107], in some cases allowing withdrawal of sulfonylurea and reduction of the insulin dose [108,109]. Hence, a few randomized trials have attempted to assess changes in insulin sensitivity comparing ACE inhibitor and placebo (Table 8) [110–117]. The results were heterogeneous, but the use of ARBs to assess insulin sensitivity seemed to show some promise, and these results were not quite as heterogeneous as those seen with ACE inhibitors. Of the seven studies shown in Table 9, five showed success in

Table 7
Prevention of type 2 diabetes mellitus by renal angiotensin aldosterone inhibition

| Study | Treatment arm: number of patients with type 2 diabetes | Treatment arm: total number of subjects | Control arm: total number of patients with diabetes mellitus | Control arm: total number of patients | Relative risk | Confidence interval | P Value favoring treatment arm |
|---|---|---|---|---|---|---|---|
| CAPP (1999) | 227 | 5184 | 280 | 5229 | 0.89 | 0.70–1.03 | NS |
| STOP-HTN-2 (1999) | 99 | 1969 | 97 | 1961 | 0.95 | 0.72–1.26 | NS |
| LIFE (2002) | 241 | 4006 | 319 | 3592 | 0.75 | 0.63–0.88 | $P = 0.001$ |
| HOPE (2001) | 102 | 2837 | 155 | 2883 | 0.66 | 0.51–0.85 | $P < 0.001$ |
| ALLHAT (2002) | 119 | 5840 | 302 | 9733 | 0.66 | 0.53–0.81 | $P < 0.001$ |
| SOLVD (2003) | 9 | 153 | 31 | 138 | 0.26 | 0.13–0.53 | $P < 0.001$ |
| ALPINE (2003) | 1 | 196 | 8 | 196 | 0.13 | 0.02–0.97 | $P = 0.03$ |
| SCOPE (2003) | 99 | 2160 | 125 | 2170 | 0.81 | 0.62–0.06 | NS |
| CHARM (2003) | 163 | 2715 | 202 | 2721 | 0.81 | 0.66–0.97 | $P < 0.001$ |
| VALUE (2004) | 690 | 7649 | 845 | 7596 | 0.77 | 0.69–0.86 | $P < 0.0001$ |

*Definitions:* ALPINE, Antihypertensive treatment and Lipid Profile in a North of Sweden Efficacy; SCOPE, Study of Cognition and Prognosis in the Elderly.

Table 8
Main randomized, placebo-controlled trials examining the effect of long-term administration of angiotensin-converting enzyme inhibitors on insulin sensitivity in patients with hypertension and/or type 2 diabetes or impaired glucose tolerance

| Reference | ACE Inhibitor, dosage | Patient characteristics | Duration of treatment | No. of patients | Blinding | Main comparator | Run-in/ washout | Insulin sensitivity assessment | Change in insulin sensitivity versus placebo |
|---|---|---|---|---|---|---|---|---|---|
| Paolisso et al, 1992 | lisinopril 20 mg/d | elderly hypertensives | 2 wks | 18 | double | placebo | 2 wks/1 wk | IVGTT | 18% increase |
| Bak et al, 1992 | perindopril 4 mg/d | hypertensives and type 2 diabetics | 6 wks | 10 | double | placebo | 2 wks/no washout | IVITT | no change |
| Santoro et al, 1993 | cliazapril 5 mg/d | hypertensives | 12 wks | 20 | open | placebo | 8 wks/NA | clamp | no change |
| Paolisso et al, 1995 | lisinopril 20 mg/d | elderly hypertensives | 8 wks | 30 | single | placebo | 3 wks/3 wks | clamp | 33% increase |
| Thurig et al, 1995 | lisinopril 20 mg/d | hypertensives | 8 wks | 24 | double | placebo | 8 wks/no washout | IVGTT | no change |
| Vuorinen-Markkola and Yki-Jarvinen, 1995 | enalapril 20–40 mg/d | hypertensives and type 2 diabetics | 4 wks | 4 | double | placebo | 4 wks/NA | clamp | 30% increase |
| Ferri et al, 1995 | captopril 25 mg bid | type 2 diabetics | 1 wk | 15 | double | placebo | none/NA | clamp | 14% increase |
| Falkner et al, 1995 | lisinopril 10–40 mg/d | black hypertensives | 12 wks | 16 | single | placebo | 8 wks/NA | clamp | 16% increase |
| Bohlen et al, 1996 | perindopril 4 mg/d | overweight hypertensives | 6 wks | 20 | double | placebo | 4 wks/NA | IVGTT | no change |
| De Mattia et al, 1996 | captopril 50 mg/d | type 2 diabetics | 10 days | 14 | double | placebo | no washout | clamp | 41% increase |
| Wiggam et al, 1998 | captopril 50 mg bid | hypertensives | 8 wks | 18 | double | placebo | 6 wks/6 wks | clamp | no change |
| Petrie et al, 2000 | trandolapril 2 mg/d | hypertensives and type 2 diabetics or persons with impaired glucose tolerance | 4 wks | 16 | double | placebo | 2 wks/2 wks | clamp | no change |

*Definitions:* IVGTT, intravenous glucose tolerance test; IVITT, intravenous insulin tolerance test; NA, not applicable.

Table 9
Main trials examining the effect of long-term therapy with angiotensin II type 1 receptor antagonists on insulin sensitivity in patients with hypertension and/or insulin resistance and/or impaired glucose tolerance

| References | AT$_1$-receptor antagonist, dosage | Patient characteristics | Duration of treatment | No. of patients | Blinding | Main comparator | Run-in/ washout | Insulin sensitivity assessment | Change in insulin sensitivity |
|---|---|---|---|---|---|---|---|---|---|
| Moan et al, 1995 | losartan 50 mg/d first 2 weeks, then 100 mg/d | hypertensive | 3–12 wks | 5 | NA | NA | 3 d washout | clamp | 30% increase |
| Laakso et al, 1996 | losartan 50 mg/d | hyperinsulinaemic and hypertensive | 12 wks | 20 | double | metoprolol 95 mg/d | 4–6 wks washout | clamp | no change |
| Paolisso et al, 1997 | losartan 50 mg/d | insulin resistant and hypertensive | 4 wks | 16 | single | placebo | 1 wk run-in | clamp | increase of NOGM |
| Fogarl et al, 1998 | losartan 50 mg/d | overweight | 6 wks/6 wks | 28 | double, crossover | perindopril 4 mg/d | 6 wks washout | clamp | ACE I improves insulin resistance |
| Fogarl et al, 1998 | losartan 50 mg/d | hypertensive | 6 wks | 25 | double, crossover | lisinopril 20 mg/d | 4 wks washout | clamp | ACE I improves insulin resistance |
| Trendwalker et al, 1998 | candesartan cilexetil 8–16 mg/d | hypertensive and type 2 diabetics | 12 wks | 161 | double | placebo | 4 wks run-in | serum HbA$_{1c}$, glycemia and lipid profile | no change |
| Higashiura et al, 1999 | candesartan | hypertensive | 2 wks | 8 | NA | NA | 2 wks run-in | clamp | increase |

*Definitions:* HbA$_{1c}$, predominant glycosylated hemoglobin; NA, not applicable; NOGM, nonoxidative metabolism.

improving insulin sensitivity [118–124]. Several factors make the results of these trials using ACE inhibitors or ARBs less robust overall. Different choice of experimental models, target molecules, doses, and route of administration may all have contributed to the conflicting results. In addition, the measure of insulin resistance itself is fraught with problems because of its sensitivity, specificity, positive and negative predictive values, reproducibility, discrimination, and calibration. The parameters used in evaluating glucose homeostasis are not always equivalent or comparable. Clearly, there is a need to improve the modeling technique by using refined methods of quantifying insulin resistance to predict more accurately the likelihood of developing diabetes and cardiovascular disease [125]. At present, metabolic syndrome variables may well be the best predictors for evaluating the likelihood of coronary artery disease.

## Summary

The role of the RAAS in development and maintenance of blood pressure is well established. In addition, the deleterious effects of angiotensin II on the heart, vasculature, and kidneys have been clearly defined. There seems to be a close relationship between endothelial dysfunction, insulin resistance (a precursor to diabetes and coronary artery disease) and angiotensin II. The signaling pathways for insulin in the vascular wall interacts with the angiotensin signaling, giving rise to potential mechanisms for development of diabetes and resulting harmful effects. A large number of clinical trials using ACE inhibitors or ARBs have shown significant reduction in secondary endpoints in the development of new onset of diabetes. Ongoing prospective studies involving ARBs (eg, the Nateglinide and Valsartan Impaired Glucose Tolerance Outcomes Research trial) and ACE inhibitors (eg, the Diabetes Reduction Assessment with Ramipril and Rosiglitazone Medication trial) are testing the ability of certain agents to prevent type 2 diabetes [125]. In the meantime, it is important to recognize insulin resistance and metabolic syndrome as entities that increase the risk for cardiovascular disease. In addition to lifestyle modifications, managing endothelial dysfunction and protecting the vasculature will help prevent diabetes and cardiovascular disease.

## References

[1] Eyre H, Kahn R, Robertson RM, the ACS/ADA/AHA Collaborative Writing Committee. Preventing cancer, cardiovascular disease, and diabetes: a common agenda for the American Cancer Society, the American Diabetes Association, and the American Heart Association. Stroke August 2004;35: 1999–2010.

[2] Chin MH, Zhang JX, Merrell K. Diabetes in the African-American Medicare population. Morbidity, quality of care, and resource utilization. Diabetes Care 1998;21:1090–5.

[3] McFarlane SI, Jacober SJ, Winer N, et al. Control of cardiovascular risk factors in patients with diabetes and hypertension at urban academic medical centers. Diabetes Care 2002;25:718–23.

[4] McVea K, Crabtree BF, Medder JD, et al. An ounce of prevention? Evaluation of the "Put Prevention into Practice" program. J Fam Pract 1996; 43:361–9.

[5] Centers for Disease Control and Prevention. National diabetes fact sheet: general information and national estimates on diabetes in the United States, 2003. Atlanta (GA): US Department of Human Services, Centers for Disease Control and Prevention; 2003. Available at: www.cdc.gov/diabetes/pubs/factsheet.htm. Accessed February 24, 2004.

[6] Narayan KM, Boyle JP, Thompson TJ, et al. Lifetime risk for diabetes mellitus in the United States. JAMA 2003;290:1884–90.

[7] Steinberger J, Daniels SR. Obesity, insulin resistance, diabetes, and cardiovascular risk in children: an American Heart Association scientific statement from the Atherosclerosis, Hypertension, and Obesity in the Young Committee (Council on Cardiovascular Disease in the Young) and the Diabetes Committee (Council on Nutrition, Physical Activity, and Metabolism). Circulation 2003;107: 1448–53.

[8] Sowers JR. Obesity as a cardiovascular risk factor. Am J Med 2003;115(Suppl 8A):37S–41S.

[9] Executive summary of the third report of the National Cholesterol Education Program (NCEP) Expert Panel on Detection, Evaluation and Treatment of High Blood Cholesterol in Adults (Adult Treatment Panel III). JAMA 2001;285: 2486–97.

[10] Harris MI, Flegal KM, Cowie CC, et al. Prevalence of diabetes, impaired fasting glucose, and impaired glucose tolerance in US adults. The Third National Health and Nutrition Examination Survey, 1988–1994. Diabetes Care 1998;21: 518–24.

[11] Park J, Edington DW. Application of a prediction model for identification of individuals at diabetic risk. Methods Inf Med 2004;43:273–81.

[12] Jarrett RJ, Keen H, Fuller JH, et al. Worsening to diabetes in men with impaired glucose tolerance

("borderline diabetes"). Diabetologia 1979;16: 25–30.

[13] Sartor G, Schersten B, Carlstrom S, et al. Ten-year follow-up of subjects with impaired glucose tolerance: prevention of diabetes by tolbutamide and diet regulation. Diabetes 1980;29:41–9.

[14] Pan XR, Li GW, Hu YH, et al. Effects of diet and exercise in preventing NIDDM in people with impaired glucose tolerance. The Da Qing IGT and Diabetes Study. Diabetes Care 1997;20: 537–44.

[15] Tuomilehto J, Geboers J, Salonen JT, et al. Decline in cardiovascular mortality in North Karelia and other parts of Finland. BMJ 1986;293: 1068–71.

[16] Knowler WC, Barrett-Connor E, Fowler SE, et al. Reduction in the incidence of type 2 diabetes with lifestyle intervention or metformin. N Engl J Med 2002;346:393–403.

[17] Klein S, Sheard NF, Pi-Sunyer X, et al. Weight management through lifestyle modification for the prevention and management of type 2 diabetes: rationale and strategies. Diabetes Care 2004;27(8): 2067–73.

[18] Zimmet P, Shaw J, Alberti KGMM. Preventing type 2 diabetes and the dysmetabolic syndrome in the real world: a realistic view. Diabet Med 2003; 20:693–702.

[19] Rosenson RS, Reasner CA. Therapeutic approaches in the prevention of cardiovascular disease in metabolic syndrome and in patients with type 2 diabetes. Curr Opin Cardiol 2004;19:480–7.

[20] Bates B, Templeton A, Achter P, et al. What does "a gene for heart disease" mean? A focus group study of public understandings of genetic risk factors. Am J Med Genet 2003;119A:156–61.

[21] Wing R, Venditti E, Jakcic J, et al. Lifestyle intervention in overweight individuals with a family history of diabetes. Diabetes Care 1998;21:350–9.

[22] Zimmet P, Shaw J, Alberti KGMM. Preventing Type 2 diabetes and the dysmetabolic syndrome in the real world: a realistic view. Diabet Med 2003;20:693–702.

[23] The CONSENSUS Trial Study Group. Effects of enalapril on mortality in severe congestive heart failure. Results of the Cooperative North Scandinavian Enalapril Survival Study (CONSENSUS). N Engl J Med 1987;316:1429–35.

[24] Garg R, Yusuf S. Overview of randomized trials of angiotensin-converting enzyme inhibitors on mortality and morbidity in patients with heart failure. Collaborative Group on ACE Inhibitor Trials. JAMA 1995;273:1450–6.

[25] Flather MD, Yusuf S, Kober L, et al. Long-term ACE-inhibitor therapy in patients with heart failure or left-ventricular dysfunction: a systematic overview of data from individual patients. ACE-Inhibitor Myocardial Infarction Collaborative Group. Lancet 2000;355:1575–81.

[26] The Acute Infarction Ramipril Efficacy (AIRE) Study Investigators. Effect of ramipril on mortality and morbidity of survivors of acute myocardial infarction with clinical evidence of heart failure. Lancet 1993;342:821–8.

[27] ACE Inhibitor Myocardial Infarction Collaborative Group. Indications for ACE inhibitors in the early treatment of acute myocardial infarction: systematic overview of individual data from 100,000 patients in randomized trials. Circulation 1998;97: 2202–12.

[28] Honan MB, Harrell FE Jr, Reimer KA, et al. Cardiac rupture, mortality and the timing of thrombolytic therapy: a meta-analysis. J Am Coll Cardiol 1990;16:359–67.

[29] Yusuf S, Sleight P, Pogue J, et al. Effects of an angiotensin-converting-enzyme inhibitor, ramipril, on cardiovascular events in high-risk patients. The Heart Outcomes Prevention Evaluation Study Investigators. N Engl J Med 2000;342:145–53.

[30] Lonn E, Yusuf S, Dzavik V, et al. Effects of ramipril and vitamin E on atherosclerosis: the Study to Evaluate Carotid Ultrasound Changes in Patients Treated with Ramipril and Vitamin E (SECURE). Circulation 2001;103:919–25.

[31] Lonn EM, Shaishkoleslami R, Yi Q, et al. Effects of ramipril on left ventricular mass and function in normotensive, high-risk patients with normal ejection fraction. A substudy of HOPE. J Am Coll Cardiol 2001;37(Suppl 2A):165A.

[32] Yusuf S. From the Heart Outcomes Prevention Evaluation Study to Ongoing Telmisartan Alone and in Combination with Ramipril Global Endpoint Trial and the Telmisartan Randomized Assessment Study in Angiotensin-Converting Enzyme Inhibitor Intolerant Patients with Cardiovascular Disease: challenges in improving prognosis. Am J Cardiol 2002;89(Suppl):18A–26A.

[33] Dahlof B, Devereux RB, Kjeldsen SE, et al. Cardiovascular morbidity and mortality in the Losartan Intervention for Endpoint reduction in hypertension study (LIFE): a randomized trial against atenolol. Lancet 2002;359:995–1003.

[34] Julius S, Kjeldsen SE, Weber M, et al, for the VALUE trial group. Outcomes in hypertensive patients at high cardiovascular risk treated with regimens based on valsartan or amlodipine: the VALUE randomized trial. Lancet 2004;363(9426):2022–31.

[35] Lewis EJ, Hunsicker LG, Clarke WR, et al. Renoprotective effect of the angiotensin-receptor antagonist irbesartan in patients with nephropathy due to type 2 diabetes. N Engl J Med 2001;345(12): 851–60.

[36] Parving HH, Lehnert H, Brochner-Mortensen J, et al. The effect of irbesartan on the development of diabetic nephropathy in patients with type 2 diabetes. N Engl J Med 2001;345(12):870–8.

[37] Brenner BM, Cooper ME, de Zeeuw D, et al. Effects of losartan on renal and cardiovascular

outcomes in patients with type 2 diabetes and nephropathy. N Engl J Med 2001;345(12):861–9.

[38] Dickstein K, Kjekshus J. Steering Committee of the OPTIMAAL Study Group. Effects of Losartan and captopril on mortality and morbidity in high-risk patients after acute myocardial infarction: the OPTIMAAL randomized trial. Optimal Trial in Myocardial Infarction with Angiotensin II Antagonist Losartan. Lancet 2002;360(9335): 752–60.

[39] Pfeffer MA, McMurray JJV, Velazquez EJ, et al, for the Valsartan in Acute Myocardial Infarction Trial Investigators. Valsartan, captopril, or both in myocardial infarction complicated by heart failure, left ventricular dysfunction, or both. N Engl J Med 2003;349:1893–906.

[40] Pitt B, Poole-Wilson PA, Segal R, et al. Effect of losartan compared with captopril on mortality in patients with symptomatic heart failure: randomized trial—the Losartan Heart Failure Survival Study ELITE II. Lancet 2000;355(9215): 1582–7.

[41] Cohn JN, Tognoni G. Valsartan Heart Failure Trial Investigators. A randomized trial of the angiotensin-receptor blocker valsartan in chronic heart failure. N Engl J Med 2001;345(23):1667–75.

[42] Pfeffer MA, Swedberg K, Granger CB, et al. CHARM Investigators and Committees. Effects of candesartan on mortality and morbidity in patients with chronic heart failure: the CHARM-Overall programme. Lancet 2003;362(9386): 759–66.

[43] Granger CB, McMurray JJ, Yusuf S, et al. CHARM Investigators and Committees. Effects of candesartan in patients with chronic heart failure and reduced left-ventricular systolic function intolerant to angiotensin-converting-enzyme inhibitors: the CHARM-Alternative Trial. Lancet 2003; 362(9386):772–6.

[44] McMurray JJ, Ostergren J, Swedberg K, et al. CHARM Investigators and Committees. Effects of candesartan in patients with chronic heart failure and reduced left ventricular systolic function taking angiotensin-converting-enzyme inhibitors: the CHARM-Added Trial. Lancet 2003;362(9386): 767–71.

[45] Yusuf S, Pfeffer MA, Swedberg K, et al. CHARM Investigators and Committees. Effects of candesartan in patients with chronic heart failure and preserved left-ventricular ejection fraction: the CHARM-Preserved Trial. Lancet 2003;362(9386): 777–81.

[46] Lucius R, Gallinat S, Busche S, et al. Beyond blood pressure: new roles for angiotensin II. Cell Mol Life Sci 1999;56:1008–19.

[47] Johnston CI, Risvanis J. Preclinical pharmacology of angiotensin II receptor antagonists: update and outstanding issues. Am J Hypertens 1997;10: 306S–10S.

[48] Chung O, Stoll M, Unger T. Physiologic and pharmacologic implications of $AT_1$ versus $AT_2$ receptors. Blood Press 1996;5(Suppl 2):47–52.

[49] Timmermans PB, Wong PC, Chiu AT, et al. Angiotensin II receptors and angiotensin II receptor antagonists. Pharmacol Rev 1993;45:205–51.

[50] Unger T, Culman J, Gohlke P. Angiotensin II receptor blockade and end-organ protection: pharmacological rationale and evidence. J Hypertens 1998;16(Suppl 7):S3–9.

[51] Drexler H, Hornig B. Endothelial dysfunction in human disease. J Mol Cell Cardiol 1999;31: 51–60.

[52] Britten MB, Zeiher AM, Schachinger V. Clinical importance of coronary endothelial vasodilator dysfunction and therapeutic options. J Intern Med 1999;245:315–27.

[53] Diet F, Pratt RE, Berry GJ, et al. Increased accumulation of tissue ACE in human atherosclerotic coronary artery disease. Circulation 1996;94: 2756–67.

[54] Shai SY, Fishel RS, Martin BM, et al. Bovine angiotensin converting enzyme cDNA cloning and regulation. Increased expression during endothelial cell growth arrest. Circ Res 1992;70: 1274–81.

[55] Fishel RS, Eisenberg S, Shai SY, et al. Glucocorticoids induce angiotensin-converting enzyme expression in vascular smooth muscle. Hypertension 1995;25:343–9.

[56] Brown NJ, Agirbasli MA, Williams GH, et al. Effect of activation and inhibition of the rennin-angiotensin system on plasma PAI-1. Hypertension 1998;32:965–71.

[57] Gainer JV, Morrow JD, Loveland A, et al. Effect of bradykinin-receptor blockade on the response to angiotensin-converting enzyme inhibitor in normotensive and hypertensive subjects. N Engl J Med 1998;339:1285–92.

[58] Hornig B, Kohler C, Drexler H. Role of bradykinin in mediating vascular effects of angiotensin-converting enzyme inhibitors in humans. Circulation 1997;95:1115–8.

[59] Lyon CJ, Law RE, Hsueh WA. Minireview: adiposity, inflammation, and atherogenesis. Endocrinology 2003;144:2195–200.

[60] Moule KS, Denton RM. Multiple signaling pathways involved in the metabolic effects of insulin. Am J Cardiol 1997;80(3):41A–9A.

[61] Nascimben L, Bothwell JH, Dominguez DY, et al. Angiotensin II stimulates insulin-independent glucose uptake in hypertrophied rat hearts [abstract]. J Hypertens 1997;15(Suppl 4):S84.

[62] Schorb W, Peeler TC, Madigan NN, et al. Angiotensin II-induced protein tyrosine phosphorylation in neonatal rat. J Biol Chem 1994;269: 19626–32.

[63] Wan J, Kurosaki T, Huant XY, et al. Tyrosine kinases in activation of the MAP-kinase cascade

by G protein-coupled receptors. Nature 1996;380: 541–4.

[64] Saad MJA, Velloso LA, Carvalho CRO. Angiotensin II induces tyrosine phosphorylation of insulin receptor substrate 1 and its association with phosphatidylinositol 3-kinase in rat heart. Biochem J 1995;310:741–4.

[65] Bernobich E, de Angelis L, Lerin C, et al. The role of the angiotensin system in cardiac glucose homeostasis. Therapeutic implications. Drugs 2002; 62(9):1295–314.

[66] Hsueh WA, Quinones MJ. Role of endothelial dysfunction in insulin resistance. Am J Cardiol 2003; 92:10J–7J.

[67] Shepherd J, Cobbe SM, Ford I, et al. Prevention of coronary heart disease with pravastatin in men with hypercholesterolemia. West of Scotland Coronary Prevention Study Group. N Engl J Med 1995;333: 1301–7.

[68] Caballero AE, Saouaf R, Lim SC, et al. The effects of troglitazone, an insulin-sensitizing agent, on the endothelial function in early and late type 2 diabetes: a placebo-controlled randomized clinical trial. Metabolism 2003;52:173–80.

[69] Avena R, Mitchell NE, Nylen ES, et al. Insulin action enhancement normalizes brachial artery vasoactivity in patients with peripheral vascular disease and occult diabetes. J Vasc Surg 1998;28: 1024–32.

[70] Saris JJ, van Dijk MA, Kroon I, et al. Functional importance of angiotensin-converting enzyme-dependent in situ angiotensin II generation in the human forearm. Hypertension 2000;35:764–8.

[71] Lyons D, Webster J, Benjamin N. Effect of enalapril and quinapril on forearm vascular ACE in man. Eur J Clin Pharmacol 1997;51:373–8.

[72] Padmanabhan N, Jardine AG, McGrath JC, et al. Angiotensin-converting enzyme-independent contraction to angiotensin I in human resistance arteries. Circulation 1999;99:2914–20.

[73] Hornig B, Arakawa N, Haussmann D, et al. Differential effects of quinaprilat and enalapril on endothelial function of conduit arteries in patients with chronic heart failure. Circulation 1998 Dec 22–29; 98(25):2842–8.

[74] Prasad A, Husain S, Quyyumi AA. Effect of enalapril on nitric oxide activity in coronary artery disease. Am J Cardiol 1999;84:1–6.

[75] Mancini GB, Henry GC, Macaya C, et al. Angiotensin-converting enzyme inhibition with quinapril improves endothelial vasomotor dysfunction in patients with coronary artery disease. The TREND (Trial on Reversing ENdothelial Dysfunction) Study. Circulation 1996 Sep 15;94(6):1490.

[76] Anderson TJ, Elstein E, Haber H, et al. Comparative study of ACE-inhibition, angiotensin II antagonism, and calcium channel blockade on flow-mediated vasodilation in patients with coronary disease (BANFF study). J Am Coll Cardiol 2000;35:60–6.

[77] Oosterga M, Voors AA, Buikema H, et al. Angiotensin II formation in human vasculature after chronic ACE inhibition: a prospective, randomized, placebo-controlled study. QUO VADIS Investigators. Cardiovasc Drugs Ther 2000;14: 55–60.

[78] Reaven GM. Syndrome X. Clinical Diabetes 1994; 12:32–6.

[79] Haffner SM, Valdez RA, Hazuda HP, et al. Prospective analysis of the insulin-resistance syndrome (syndrome X). Diabetes 1992;41:715–22.

[80] Mykkanen L, Kuusisto J, Pyorala K, et al. Cardiovascular disease risk factors as predictors on type 2 (non-insulin-dependent) diabetes mellitus in elderly subjects. Diabetologia 1993;36:553–9.

[81] Lakka HM, Laaksonen D, Lakka T, et al. The MetS and total cardiovascular mortality in middle-aged men. JAMA 2002;228:2709–16.

[82] Isomaa B, Henricsson M, Almgren P, et al. The MetS influences the risk of chronic complications in patients with type II diabetes. Diabetologia 2001;44:1148–54.

[83] Alberti KG. The clinical implications of impaired glucose tolerance. Diabet Med 1996;13:927–37.

[84] Edelstein SL, Knowler WC, Bain RP, et al. Predictors of progression from impaired glucose tolerance of NIDDM: an analysis of six prospective studies. Diabetes 1997;46:701–10.

[85] Lorenzo C, Okoloise M, Williams K, et al. The MetS as predictor of type 2 diabetes. Diabetes Care 2003;26:3153–9.

[86] Snehalatha C, Mukesh B, Simon M, et al. Plasma adiponectin is an independent predictor of type 2 diabetes in Asian Indians. Diabetes Care 2003; 26(12):3226.

[87] Farquhar JW, Fortmann SP, Flora JA, et al. Effects of communitywide education on cardiovascular disease risk factors. The Stanford Five-City Project. JAMA 1990;264:359–65.

[88] Luepker RV, Murray DM, Jacobs DR Jr, et al. Community education for cardiovascular disease prevention: risk factor changes in the Minnesota Heart Health Program. Am J Public Health 1994; 84:1383–93.

[89] Younis N, Soran H, Farook S. The prevention of type 2 diabetes mellitus: recent advances. Q J Med 2004;97:451–5.

[90] Lindstrom J, Louheranta A, Mannelin M, et al. National Public Health Institute, Diabetes and Genetic Epidemiologic Unit, FI-00300 Helsinki, Finland. The Finnish Diabetes Prevention Study (DPS). Diabetes Care 2003;26(12):3230.

[91] Watanabe M, Yamaoka K, Yokotsuka M, et al. Randomized controlled trial of a new dietary education program to prevent type 2 diabetes in a high-risk group of Japanese male workers. Diabetes Care 2003;26(12):3209.

[92] Keen H, Jarrett RJ, McCartney P, et al. The ten-year follow-up of the Bedford survey (1962–1972):

glucose tolerance and diabetes. Diabetologia 1982; 22:73–8.

[93] Tuomilehto J, Lindstrom J, Eriksson JG, et al. Prevention of type 2 diabetes mellitus by changes in lifestyle among subjects with impaired glucose tolerance. N Engl J Med 2001;344:1343–50.

[94] Jacques CH, Jones RL. Problems encountered by primary care physicians in the care of patients with diabetes. Arch Fam Med 1993;2:739–41.

[95] Shintani TT, Hughes CK, Beckham S, et al. Obesity and cardiovascular risk intervention through the ad libitum feeding of traditional Hawaiian diet. Am J Clin Nutr 1991;53:1647S–51S.

[96] Yusuf S, Gerstein H, Hoogwerf B, et al, for the HOPE Study Investigators. Ramipril and the development of diabetes. JAMA 2001;286(15): 1882–5.

[97] The ALLHAT Officers and Coordinators for the ALLHAT Collaborative Research Group. Major outcomes in high-risk hypertensive patients randomized to angiotensin-converting enzyme inhibitor or calcium channel blocker vs diuretic: the Antihypertensive and Lipid-Lowering Treatment to Prevent Heart Attack Trial (ALLHAT). JAMA 2002;288(23):2981–97.

[98] Lindholm LH, Ibsen H, Dahlof B, et al. Cardiovascular morbidity and mortality in patients with diabetes in the Losartan Intervention For Endpoint reduction in hypertension study (LIFE): a randomized trial against atenolol. Lancet 2002;359: 1004–10.

[99] Lindholm LH, Persson M, Alaupovic P, et al. Metabolic outcome during 1 year in newly detected hypertensives: results of the Antihypertensive Treatment and Lipid Profile in a North of Sweden Efficacy Evaluation (ALPINE) study. J Hypertens 2003;21(8):1563–74.

[100] Papademetriou V, Farsang C, Elmfeldt D, et al. Study on Cognition and Prognosis in the Elderly study group. Stroke prevention with the angiotensin II type 1-receptor blocker candesartan in elderly patients with isolated systolic hypertension: the Study on Cognition and Prognosis in the Elderly (SCOPE). J Am Coll Cardiol 2004; 44(6):1175–80.

[101] Ekbom T, Linjer E, Hedner T, et al. Cardiovascular events in elderly patients with isolated systolic hypertension. A subgroup analysis of treatment strategies in STOP-Hypertension-2. Blood Press 2004; 13(3):137–41.

[102] The Captopril Prevention Project (CAPP) Study Group. Effect of angiotensin-converting enzyme inhibition compared with conventional therapy on cardiovascular morbidity and mortality in hypertension: the Captopril Prevention Project (CAPP) randomized trial. Curr Hypertens Rep 1999;1(6): 466–7.

[103] Mazzone T. Strategies in ongoing clinical trials to reduce cardiovascular disease in patients with diabetic mellitus and insulin resistance. Am J Cardiol 2004;93(11A):27C–31C.

[104] Drexler AJ. Lessons learned from landmark trials of type 2 diabetes mellitus and potential applications to clinical practice [special issue]. Postgrad Med 2003;15–26.

[105] Aranda JM Jr, Conti R. Angiotensin II blockade: a therapeutic strategy with wide applications. Clin Cardiol 2003;26:500–2.

[106] White M, Racine N, Ducharme A, et al. Therapeutic potential of angiotensin II receptor antagonists. Expert Opin Investig Drugs 2001;10(9): 1687–701.

[107] Paolisso G, Gambardella A, Verza M, et al. ACE inhibition improves insulin-sensitivity in aged insulin-resistant hypertensive patients. J Hum Hypertens 1992;6(3):175–9.

[108] De Mattia G, Ferri C, Laurenti O, et al. Circulating catecholamines and metabolic effects of captopril in NIDDM patients. Diabetes Care 1996;19(3): 226–30.

[109] Wiggam MI, Hunter SJ, Atkinson AB, et al. Captopril does not improve insulin action in essential hypertension: a double-blind placebo-controlled study. J Hypertens 1998;16(11):1651–7.

[110] Bak JF, Gerdes LU, Sorenson NS, et al. Effects of perindopril on insulin sensitivity and plasma lipid profile in hypertensive non-insulin-dependent diabetic patients. Am J Med 1992;92(4B):69S–72S.

[111] Santoro D, Galvan AQ, Natali A, et al. Some metabolic aspects of essential hypertension and its treatment. Am J Med 1993;94(4A):32S–9S.

[112] Paolisso G, Balbi V, Gambardella A, et al. Lisinopril administration improves insulin action in aged patients with hypertension. J Hum Hypertens 1995; 9(7):541–6.

[113] Thurig C, Bohlen L, Schneider M, et al. Lisinopril is neutral to insulin sensitivity and serum lipoproteins in essential hypertensive patients. Eur J Clin Pharmacol 1995;49(1–2):21–6.

[114] Vuorinen-Markolla H, Yki-Jarvinen H. Antihypertensive therapy with Enalapril improves glucose storage and insulin sensitivity in hypertensive patients with non-insulin-dependent diabetes mellitus. Metabolism 1995;44(1):85–9.

[115] Falkner B, Canessa M, Anzalone D. Effect of angiotensin converting enzyme inhibitor (lisinopril) on insulin sensitivity and sodium transport in mild hypertension. Am J Hypertens 1995;8(5 Pt 1): 454–60.

[116] Bohlen L, Bienz R, Doser M, et al. Metabolic neutrality of perindopril: focus on insulin sensitivity in overweight patients with essential hypertension. J Cardiovasc Pharmacol 1996;27(6):770–6.

[117] Petrie JR, Morris AD, Ueda S, et al. Trandopril does not improve insulin sensitivity in patients with hypertension and type 2 diabetes: a double-blind, placebo-controlled crossover trial. J Clin Endocrinol Metab 2000;85(5):1882–9.

[118] Moan A, Hoieggen A, Nordby G, et al. Effects of losartan on insulin sensitivity in severe hypertension: connection with sympathetic nervous system activity? J Hum Hypertens 1995;9:S45–50.

[119] Laasko M, Karjalainen L, Lempiainen-Kuosa P. Effects of losartan on insulin sensitivity in hypertensive subjects. Hypertension 1996;28:392–6.

[120] Paolisso G, Tagliamonte MR, Gambardella A, et al. Losartan mediated improvement in insulin action is mainly due to a non-oxidative glucose metabolism and blood flow in insulin-resistant hypertensive patients. J Hum Hypertens 1997;11(5):307–12.

[121] Fogari R, Zopp A, Lazzari P, et al. ACE-inhibition but not angiotensin II antagonism reduces plasma fibrinogen and insulin resistance in overweight hypertensive patients. J Cardiovasc Pharmacol 1998; 32(4):616–20.

[122] Fogari R, Zoppi A, Corradi L, et al. Comparative effects of lisinopril and losartan on insulin sensitivity in the treatment of non-diabetic hypertensive patients. Br J Clin Pharmacol 1998;46:467–71.

[123] Trenkwalder P, Dahl K, Lehtovirta M, et al. Antihypertensive treatment with candesartan cilexitil does not affect glucose homeostasis or serum lipid profile in patients with mild hypertension and type II diabetes. Blood Press 1998;7(3): 170–5.

[124] Higashiura K, Ura N, Miyazaki Y, et al. Effects of angiotensin II receptor antagonist, candesartan cilexitil, on insulin resistance and pressor mechanisms in essential hypertension. J Hum Hypertens 1999; 13(Suppl. 1):S71–4.

[125] Evans M, McEwan P, Peters JR, et al. Should we routinely measure a proxy for insulin resistance as well as improve our modeling techniques to better predict the likelihood of coronary heart disease in people with type 2 diabetes? For debate. Diabetes Obes Metab 2004;6:299–307.

CARDIOLOGY
CLINICS

Cardiol Clin 23 (2005) 185–191

# Percutaneous Coronary Intervention Versus Coronary Artery Bypass Grafting in Diabetic Patients

Debabrata Mukherjee, MD, MS, FACC

*Division of Cardiovascular Medicine, University of Kentucky, 900 S. Limestone Street, 326 Wethington Building, Lexington, KY 40536-0200, USA*

### Coronary revascularization in diabetics

Diabetic patients who have coronary artery disease have significantly worse long-term outcomes compared with nondiabetic patients. The reasons for this are complex but relate, in part, to more extensive atherosclerosis, an increased risk of thrombosis, overexpression of mitogenic cytokines, higher oxidative stress, glycated end products, larger and more activated platelets, and more rapid progression of disease. Patients who have diabetes experience higher perioperative mortality rates compared with nondiabetics who undergo bypass surgery (CABG) [1,2] or percutaneous coronary intervention (PCI) [3,4]. Although outcomes after revascularization in diabetics are worse after either modality, CABG seems to be preferable to PCI in most patients who have multi-vessel disease (Fig. 1).

### Percutaneous coronary intervention versus bypass surgery as revascularization modality

The Bypass Angioplasty Revascularization Investigation (BARI), reported that in diabetic patients who had symptomatic multi-vessel disease, CABG resulted in a significantly better outcome compared with PCI at 5 years [5] and at 7 years [6]. Among treated diabetic patients, 5-year survival was 80.6% for the CABG group and 65.5% for the percutaneous transluminal coronary angioplasty (PTCA) group ($P = 0.003$). The benefit was confined largely to patients who

had more severe multi-vessel disease and those who received left internal mammary artery (LIMA) bypass grafts; no benefit was seen in patients who received only saphenous vein grafts. In the BARI registry, with revascularization modality primarily based on physician judgement, the all-cause mortality was 14.4% for PTCA versus 14.9% for CABG ($P = 0.86$; relative risk [RR] $= 1.10$), with corresponding cardiac mortality rates of 7.5% and 6.0%, respectively ($P = 0.73$; RR $= 1.07$) [7]. The higher mortality with PCI in diabetics was confirmed in the 8-year follow-up of the Emory Angioplasty versus Surgery Trial (EAST) [8] and Coronary Angioplasty versus Bypass Revascularization Investigation (CABRI Trial) [9]. In the EAST trial there were 59 treated diabetic patients—30 in the surgical group and 29 in the angioplasty group. At 3 years, the survival was similar (surgery 90%, angioplasty 93.1%); this also was similar to the patients without treated diabetes. In the extended follow-up, after 5 years the curves began to diverge; by 8 years, there was a trend toward improved survival with CABG in the diabetic group (surgical survival 75.5%, angioplasty 60.1%, $P = 0.23$) [8]. In the CABRI population, diabetics who were randomized to PCI and those who were randomized to CABG had higher mortality than respective nondiabetics. Among diabetics, there was a strong trend toward higher mortality with PCI compared with CABG (RR, 1.81; 95% confidence interval [CI], 0.80–4.08) [9]. In the Mid America Heart Institute single-center registry of diabetic patients who underwent revascularization, freedom from death (30% versus 37%; $P = 0.08$), myocardial infarction, and subsequent revascularization during long-term follow-up was superior with CABG

Supported in part by a grant from the Mardigian Foundation.

*E-mail address:* mukherjee@uky.edu

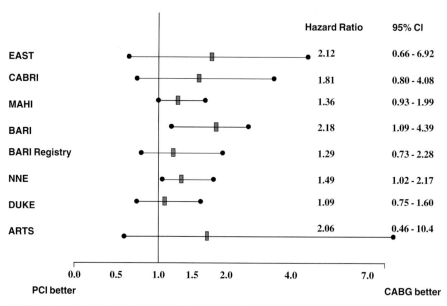

Fig. 1. Mortality in diabetics undergoing revascularization. Estimated hazard ratios (and 95% confidence intervals) for mortality at follow-up for initial PCI compared with CABG among diabetic patients with multi-vessel disease. ARTS, Arterial Revascularization Therapy Study; BARI, Bypass-Angioplasty Revascularization Investigation; CABG, coronary artery bypass grafting; CABRI, Coronary Angioplasty versus Bypass Revascularization Investigation; DUKE, Duke University Medical Center Registry; EAST, Emory Angioplasty versus Surgery Trial; MAHI, Mid America Heart Institute; NNE, Northern New England database study; PCI, percutaneous coronary intervention.

compared with angioplasty [10]. In the Duke University Medical Center registry, diabetes was associated with a worse long-term outcome after PCI and CABG in patients who had multi-vessel coronary artery disease, with no significant difference in outcomes between PCI and CABG [11].

These trials were conducted before the introduction of coronary stenting and adjunctive therapies, such as glycoprotein (GP) IIb/IIIa drugs and prolonged dual antiplatelet therapy. The recent results of the Arterial Revascularization Therapy Study (ARTS Trial) were the first to specifically address the role of coronary stenting versus CABG in diabetic patients who had multi-vessel disease [12]. In this study, 1205 patients who had multi-vessel disease were randomized to stent placement or CABG. Of the 1205 patients, 208 had diabetes (defined as a history of diabetes mellitus on oral hypoglycemic agents or insulin) at entry. Both groups had an average of 2.7 lesions treated and 89% of the surgical patients received a LIMA graft. In-hospital events were similar between the groups; at 1 year the CABG group and PCI group had similar death rates (3.1% versus 6.3%, $P = 0.40$) and myocardial infarction rates (3.1% versus 6.3%, $P = 0.40$). Patients who underwent CABG had a significantly lower repeat

revascularization rate (3.1% versus 22%, $P < 0.001$). Overall event-free survival was 84.4% for the CABG group and 63.4% for the stent group ($P < 0.001$). This study emphasized the poor outcome of diabetic patients after revascularization and the value of bypass surgery with LIMA graft in patients who have diabetes and multi-vessel disease. The study does not mean, however, that coronary stents in diabetics are not beneficial. Numerous studies have shown that stents decreased restenosis in diabetics as well as in non-diabetics [13]. The BARI Registry included all BARI patients who were eligible for randomization, but who refused. This group was followed to the same extent as were the BARI randomized patients. Within this group, the outcome of the treated diabetic patients who received PCI was equivalent to those who received CABG [7]. Patients who received CABG had more extensive multi-vessel disease and more diffuse disease than did the patients who underwent angioplasty, whereas the patients who underwent angioplasty had more discrete two-vessel disease. The decision to choose PCI or CABG was left to the discretion of the treating physician. The Bypass Angioplasty Revascularization Investigation 2 Diabetes (BARI 2D) Trial that is comparing revascularization with no revascularization in asymptomatic or mildly symptomatic patients who have diabetes and coronary disease will allow either form of revascularization; physician judgment seems to select patients appropriately for both revascularization modalities. A major limitation of the ARTS trial is that most patients did not receive GP IIb/IIIa drugs. In contemporary PCI, the role of concomitant GP IIb/IIIa inhibition is established firmly. The Evaluation of IIb/IIIa Platelet Inhibitor for Stenting (EPISTENT) study demonstrated reduced mortality in patients who received stents who were randomized to abciximab instead of placebo [14]. The mortality benefit of GP IIb/IIIa blockade was magnified in diabetic patients [15]. Furthermore, in a pooled analysis of abciximab in PCI trials, diabetic patients who were randomized to abciximab demonstrated mortality rates that were similar to those in nondiabetics patients who received placebo [16]. Thus, abciximab administration essentially converted the risk of death for the diabetic to that of a nondiabetic patient. This mortality benefit is particularly marked in the subset of diabetics who has multi-vessel disease [17]. Additionally, the EPISTENT trial showed that abciximab reduced clinical and angiographic restenosis in diabetic patients [15]. Restenosis, especially in its occlusive form, is a major determinant of long-term mortality in diabetic patients after coronary balloon angioplasty [18]; any benefit of abciximab in reducing restenosis consequently may translate to a survival advantage. Thus, GP IIb/IIIa blockade could have changed the results of the BARI and the ARTS trial dramatically in terms of restenosis and mortality; this concept needs to be tested prospectively.

The beneficial effects of long-term clopidogrel on patients who underwent PCI was evaluated in the PCI-Clopidogrel in Unstable angina to prevent Recurrent Events trial (PCI CURE) [19] and the Clopidogrel for Reduction of Events During Observation trial (CREDO) [20]. The PCI CURE trial demonstrated that in patients who had acute coronary syndrome undergoing PCI, longer-term administration of clopidogrel therapy (for a mean period of 8 months) reduced the risk of cardiovascular death or myocardial infarction by about a third, compared with placebo [19]. In more elective nonacute coronary patients, the CREDO trial demonstrated that continuation of dual antiplatelet therapy with clopidogrel and aspirin for at least 1 year, instead of the current standard of 2 to 4 weeks, led to a statistically and clinically significant reduction in major thrombotic events with a 26.9% relative reduction in the combined risk of death, myocardial infarction, or stroke (95% CI, 3.9%–44.4%; $P = 0.02$; absolute reduction, 3%) [20]. Prolonged dual antiplatelet therapy with aspirin plus clopidogrel also could be applicable and beneficial after CABG [21]. Other evidence-based therapies, such as β-blockers, continue to be underused in diabetic patients who undergo revascularization and may significantly improve outcomes after CABG [22] and PCI [23]. One should also keep in mind the potentially debilitating effects of central nervous system function disturbance and dramatic decrease in neurocognitive function post-CABG [24], which would give PCI the edge.

*Repeat revascularization in diabetic patients who had previous bypass surgery*

Diabetic patients who have recurrent disease after CBG have three options: medical therapy, PCI, or redo CABG. There is significant uncertainty and controversy concerning the choice of revascularization for diabetic patients who have had previous CABG. One study evaluated short- and long-term outcomes of diabetic patients who underwent repeat CABG or PCI after initial CABG [25]. In-hospital mortality was greater for redo CABG; however, differences in long-term mortality were not significant (10-year mortality, 68% PCI versus 74% CABG; $P = 0.14$). Overall, the decision to proceed with PCI or redo CABG in diabetic patients after first coronary surgery should take into account the higher initial mortality of redo CABG and the similar long-term results with either revascularization modality. For some patients, this may suggest that it is appropriate to proceed with an initial strategy of PCI. The choice of redo CABG should be based on individual patient characteristics, such as the ability to provide new arterial conduits or the presence of unprotected native left main disease or long segments of severe diffuse disease in the native vessels. Individual physicians often make revascularization decisions for these patients based on angiographic evaluation that is tailored to each patient. Evidence that CABG offers better outcome than PCI for a first revascularization procedure in diabetic patients who have multi-vessel disease cannot be extrapolated to diabetic patients who had previous CABG. Rather, choices must be based on clinical and angiographic evaluation of each patient and patient preference.

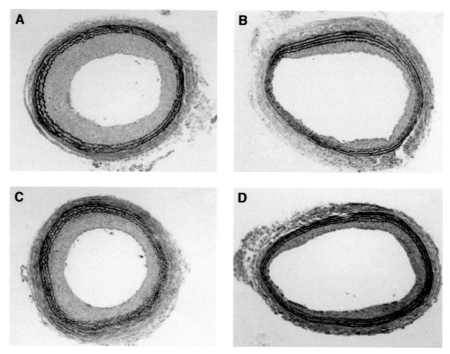

Fig. 2. Suppression of neointimal hyperplasia by soluble receptor for advanced glycation end products (sRAGE) (Van Gieson, 10×) Light miscroscopy cross-sections of injured arteries. (*A*) Zucker diabetic rat control group showing extensive neointimal hyperplasia with smaller luminal area. (*B*) sRAGE-treated diabetic rat showing reduced neointimal hyperplasia with larger luminal area. (*C*) Zucker nondiabetic rat control group showing extensive neointimal hyperplasia with smaller luminal area. (*D*) sRAGE-treated nondiabetic rat showing reduced neointimal hyperplasia with larger luminal area. (*Adapted from* Zhou Z, Wang K, Penn MS, Marso SP, Lauer MA, Forudi F, et al. Receptor for AGE (RAGE) mediates neointimal formation in response to arterial injury. Circulation 2003;107(17):2238–43; with permission.)

*Bypass Angioplasty Revascularization Investigation 2 Diabetes Trial*

Patients who have diabetes respond less favorably to PCI or CABG compared with nondiabetic patients. The recent advent of insulin sensitizers enables clinicians to target treatment of insulin resistance, hyperglycemia, and dyslipidemia. These considerations led to the initiation of the BARI 2D trial [26]. It is designed to determine whether treatment that is targeted to attenuate insulin resistance can arrest or retard progression of coronary artery disease better than treatment that is targeted to the same level of glycemic control with an insulin-providing approach. It also is designed to determine whether early revascularization reduces mortality and morbidity in patients who have type 2 diabetes whose cardiac symptoms are mild and stable. The primary objective of the BARI 2D trial is to test simultaneously, with the use of a 2×2 factorial design, two clinically-discrete hypotheses regarding the efficacy of treatment in patients who have type 2 diabetes and stable coronary artery disease who may be candidates for coronary revascularization [26].

One hypothesis that is being tested in the trial compares two modalities of diabetes treatment: (1) pharmacologic therapy that is designed to induce glycemic and metabolic control by provision of endogenous or exogenous insulin and (2) pharmacologic therapies that are designed to induce comparable glycemic and metabolic control by amelioration of insulin resistance. The target for glycemic control in both groups is reduction of hemoglobin A1C concentrations to 7.0%. The other hypothesis that is being tested in the trial is optimal treatment of the coronary artery disease. The strategies that are being compared are intensive pharmacologic management of coronary artery disease (including the use of β-blockers, angiotensin-converting enzyme inhibitors, antilipemic agents, and aspirin) and intensive pharmacologic management plus initial

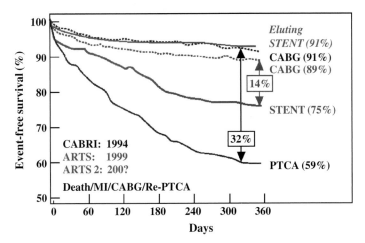

Fig. 3. Hypothetic event-free survival of a cohort of patients who had multi-vessel coronary artery disease who were treated with a rapamycin-eluting stent. This suggests a clinical outcome at 1 year that was comparable or superior to a surgical outcome. There is a large gap (32%) in event-free survival between patients who underwent bypasses and patients who were treated with conventional balloon angioplasty. This gap was reduced to 14% with the use of stents. Percentages in parenthesis denote event-free survival. CABG (89%) refers to survival in 1994. CABG (91%) refers to survival in 1999, 2000?, date for ARTS 2 result is unknown at this time. (*Adapted from* Serruys PW. ARTS I—the rapamycin eluting stent; ARTS II—the rosy prophecy. Eur Heart J 2002;23(10):757–9; with permission.)

coronary revascularization by either PCI or CABG as selected by the patient in consultation with the treating physician. Both treatment arms include lifestyle monitoring and strict management of all conventional, modifiable risk factors. Patients who are assigned to the intensive medical management arm may undergo revascularization during follow-up as clinically necessary consistent with the rationale for allowing attending physician/patient choice of CABG or PCI that was delineated above [26]. The results of BARI 2D may help to define optimal management of diabetic patients who have coronary artery disease.

## Emerging therapies

Several emerging therapies may improve clinical outcomes after coronary revascularization in diabetics. Drug-coated stents, currently being tested in clinical trials, ultimately could reduce restenosis rates to an unprecedented low level. The report from the randomized study with the sirolimus coated Bx velocity balloon expandable stent in the treatment of patients with de novo native coronary artery lesions. Trial suggested that drug-eluting stents may reduce restenosis dramatically [27]. In this trial, none of the patients in the sirolimus-stent group (as compared with 26.6% of those in the standard-stent group) had

restenosis of 50% or more of the luminal diameter ($P < 0.001$). During a follow-up period of up to 1 year, the overall rate of major cardiac events was 5.8% in the sirolimus-stent group and 28.8% in the standard-stent group ($P < 0.001$) [27]. The difference was due entirely to a higher rate of revascularization of the target vessel in the standard-stent group. In the subgroup of patients who had diabetes, 19 patients received sirolimus-eluting stents and 25 received standard stents. The minimal luminal diameter before and after stenting was similar in the two groups (0.99 mm in the sirolimus-stent group and 0.93 mm in the standard-stent group before the procedure and 2.37 and 2.36 mm afterward, respectively). At 6 months, the minimal luminal diameter was markedly larger in the sirolimus-stent group (2.29 mm versus 1.56 mm; $P < 0.001$); consequently, the late loss was smaller (0.07 mm in the sirolimus-stent group versus 0.82 mm in the standard-stent group; $P < 0.001$) and the restenosis rate was lower (0% versus 41.7%; $P = 0.002$) [27].

One must keep in mind that although a significant proportion of adverse events in diabetics is related to restenosis, there also is a significant component of rapid progression of coronary disease. This could impact outcomes adversely after PCI as compared with the CABG group, who would have vascular conduits bypassing large areas of potentially obstructable diseased coronary arteries [18]. Thus, drug-eluting stents alone may not be sufficient in reducing events during follow-up.

Recent molecular studies demonstrated a key role for the receptor for advanced glycation end products (RAGE) in modulating smooth muscle cell properties after vascular injury. It was suggested that RAGE is a logical target for suppression of untoward neointimal expansion consequent to arterial injury in diabetic patients [28]. Zhou et al [29] demonstrated that blockade of RAGE/ligand interaction significantly decreased S100-stimulated vascular smooth muscle cell (VSMC) proliferation in vitro and bromodeoxyuridine-labeled proliferating VSMC in vivo, suppressed neointimal formation, and increased luminal area in Zucker diabetic and nondiabetic rats. In the future, blockade of RAGE may have significant therapeutic potential after PCI (Fig. 2).

## Summary

Revascularization with CABG or angioplasty in diabetic patients is associated with a less favorable outcome. The value of early intervention will be assessed in the ongoing BARI 2D trial. It remains to be determined whether the widespread use of GP IIb/IIIa drugs and prolonged dual antiplatelet therapy in diabetic patients who receive stents, and possibly drug-eluting stents, will alter results significantly so that outcomes become comparable or even better than CABG (Fig. 3). It seems prudent to consider CABG with LIMA grafting in diabetic patients who have severe multi-vessel disease and to consider angioplasty in selected patients who have more discrete and less severe disease.

## References

[1] Thourani VH, Weintraub WS, Stein B, Gebhart SS, Craver JM, Jones EL, et al. Influence of diabetes mellitus on early and late outcome after coronary artery bypass grafting. Ann Thorac Surg 1999; 67(4):1045–52.

[2] Smith LR, Harrell FE Jr, Rankin JS, Califf RM, Pryor DB, Muhlbaier LH, et al. Determinants of early versus late cardiac death in patients undergoing coronary artery bypass graft surgery. Circulation 1991;84(5 Suppl):245–53.

[3] Stein B, Weintraub WS, Gebhart SP, Cohen-Bernstein CL, Grosswald R, Liberman HA, et al. Influence of diabetes mellitus on early and late outcome after percutaneous transluminal coronary angioplasty. Circulation 1995;91(4):979–89.

[4] Kip KE, Faxon DP, Detre KM, Yeh W, Kelsey SF, Currier JW. Coronary angioplasty in diabetic patients. The National Heart, Lung, and Blood Institute Percutaneous Transluminal Coronary Angioplasty Registry. Circulation 1996;94(8):1818–25.

[5] Comparison of coronary bypass surgery with angioplasty in patients with multivessel disease. The Bypass Angioplasty Revascularization Investigation (BARI) Investigators. N Engl J Med 1996;335(4): 217–25.

[6] Seven-year outcome in the Bypass Angioplasty Revascularization Investigation (BARI) by treatment and diabetic status. J Am Coll Cardiol 2000;35(5): 1122–9.

[7] Detre KM, Guo P, Holubkov R, Califf RM, Sopko G, Bach R, et al. Coronary revascularization in diabetic patients: a comparison of the randomized and observational components of the Bypass Angioplasty Revascularization Investigation (BARI). Circulation 1999;99(5):633–40.

[8] King SB III, Kosinski AS, Guyton RA, Lembo NJ, Weintraub WS. Eight-year mortality in the Emory Angioplasty versus Surgery Trial (EAST). J Am Coll Cardiol 2000;35(5):1116–21.

[9] Kurbaan AS, Bowker TJ, Ilsley CD, Sigwart U, Rickards AF. Difference in the mortality of the CABRI diabetic and nondiabetic populations and its relation to coronary artery disease and the revascularization mode. Am J Cardiol 2001;87(8): 947–50.

[10] Gum PA, O'Keefe JH Jr, Borkon AM, Spertus JA, Bateman TM, McGraw JP, et al. Bypass surgery versus coronary angioplasty for revascularization of treated diabetic patients. Circulation 1997;96 (9 Suppl):7–10.

[11] Barsness GW, Peterson ED, Ohman EM, Nelson CL, DeLong ER, Reves JG, et al. Relationship between diabetes mellitus and long-term survival after coronary bypass and angioplasty. Circulation 1997;96(8):2551–6.

[12] Serruys PW, Unger F, Sousa JE, Jatene A, Bonnier HJ, Schonberger JP, et al. Comparison of coronary-artery bypass surgery and stenting for the treatment of multivessel disease. N Engl J Med 2001;344(15):1117–24.

[13] Malenka DJ, O'Connor GT, Quinton H, Wennberg D, Robb JF, Shubrooks S, et al. Differences in outcomes between women and men associated with percutaneous transluminal coronary angioplasty. A regional prospective study of 13,061 procedures. Northern New England Cardiovascular Disease Study Group. Circulation 1996;94(9 Suppl):99–104.

[14] Topol EJ, Mark DB, Lincoff AM, Cohen E, Burton J, Kleiman N, et al. Outcomes at 1 year and economic implications of platelet glycoprotein IIb/IIIa blockade in patients undergoing coronary stenting: results from a multicentre randomised trial. EPISTENT Investigators. Evaluation of Platelet

IIb/IIIa Inhibitor for Stenting. Lancet 2003; 354(9195):2019–24.

[15] Marso SP, Lincoff AM, Ellis SG, Bhatt DL, Tanguay JF, Kleiman NS, et al. Optimizing the percutaneous interventional outcomes for patients with diabetes mellitus: results of the EPISTENT (Evaluation of platelet IIb/IIIa inhibitor for stenting trial) diabetic substudy. Circulation 1999; 1999;100(5):2477–84.

[16] Bhatt DL, Marso SP, Lincoff AM, Wolski KE, Ellis SG, Topol EJ. Abciximab reduces mortality in diabetics following percutaneous coronary intervention. J Am Coll Cardiol 2000;35(4):922–8.

[17] Bhatt D, Lincoff A, Tcheng J, Califf R, L'Allier P, Marso S, et al. The impact of abciximab on mortality after multivessel PCI: a striking effect in diabetics. J Am Coll Cardiol 2000;35:91A.

[18] Van Belle E, Ketelers R, Bauters C, Perie M, Abolmaali K, Richard F, et al. Patency of percutaneous transluminal coronary angioplasty sites at 6-month angiographic follow-up: A key determinant of survival in diabetics after coronary balloon angioplasty. Circulation 2001;103(9):1218–24.

[19] Mehta SR, Yusuf S, Peters RJ, Bertrand ME, Lewis BS, Natarajan MK, et al. Effects of pretreatment with clopidogrel and aspirin followed by long-term therapy in patients undergoing percutaneous coronary intervention: the PCI-CURE study. Lancet 2001;358(9281):527–33.

[20] Steinhubl SR, Berger PB, Mann JT III, Fry ET, DeLago A, Wilmer C, et al. Early and sustained dual oral antiplatelet therapy following percutaneous coronary intervention: a randomized controlled trial. JAMA 2002;288(19):2411–20.

[21] Bhatt DL, Chew DP, Hirsch AT, Ringleb PA, Hacke W, Topol EJ. Superiority of clopidogrel versus aspirin in patients with prior cardiac surgery. Circulation 2001;103(3):363–8.

[22] Ferguson TB Jr, Coombs LP, Peterson ED. Preoperative beta-blocker use and mortality and morbidity following CABG surgery in North America. JAMA 2002;287(17):2221–7.

[23] Mukherjee D, Smith D, Kline-Rogers E, Chetcuti S, Eagle K, Grossman P, et al. Significant mortality benefit of prior beta-blocker use in diabetic patients undergoing coronary intervention. Eur Heart J 2002;23(Suppl):317.

[24] Newman MF, Kirchner JL, Phillips-Bute B, Gaver V, Grocott H, Jones RH, et al. Longitudinal assessment of neurocognitive function after coronary-artery bypass surgery. N Engl J Med 2001;344(6):395–402.

[25] Cole JH, Jones EL, Craver JM, Guyton RA, Morris DC, Douglas JS, et al. Outcomes of repeat revascularization in diabetic patients with prior coronary surgery. J Am Coll Cardiol 2002;40(11): 1968–75.

[26] Sobel BE, Frye R, Detre KM. Burgeoning dilemmas in the management of diabetes and cardiovascular disease: rationale for the Bypass Angioplasty Revascularization Investigation 2 Diabetes (BARI 2D) Trial. Circulation 2003;107(4):636–42.

[27] Morice MC, Serruys PW, Sousa JE, Fajadet J, Ban Hayashi E, Perin M, et al. A randomized comparison of a sirolimus-eluting stent with a standard stent for coronary revascularization. N Engl J Med 2002; 346(23):1773–80.

[28] Sakaguchi T, Yan SF, Yan SD, Belov D, Rong LL, Sousa M, et al. Central role of RAGE-dependent neointimal expansion in arterial restenosis. J Clin Invest 2003;111(7):959–72.

[29] Zhou Z, Wang K, Penn MS, Marso SP, Lauer MA, Forudi F, et al. Receptor for AGE (RAGE) mediates neointimal formation in response to arterial injury. Circulation 2003; 107(17):2238–43.

CARDIOLOGY
CLINICS

Cardiol Clin 23 (2005) 193–210

# Comprehensive Risk Reduction of Cardiovascular Risk Factors in the Diabetic Patient: An Integrated Approach

Sundararajan Srikanth, MD,
Prakash Deedwania, MD, FACC, FACP, FCCP, FAHA*

*Department of Medicine, VA Central California Health Care System/University Medical Center,
University of California, San Francisco Program at Fresno,
2615 East Clinton Avenue, Fresno, CA 93703, USA*

The Egyptians recognized diabetes as a pathologic entity nearly 3500 years ago. It was noted to be a rare condition but was known to reduce longevity. The condition now defined as type 2 diabetes is seen worldwide and has reached epidemic proportions. By the year 2025, the number of individuals with diabetes mellitus in the world is expected to exceed 300 million with a prevalence of 5.4% [1]. Diabetes continues to affect a substantial proportion of adults in the United States. Data from the National Health and Nutrition Enhancement Survey 1999–2000 indicate that 8.3% of persons over the age of 20 years have either diagnosed or undiagnosed diabetes, and this percentage increases to 19.2% for persons aged more than 60 years in the United States. Men and women are affected similarly by diabetes [2]. In 1999–2000, an additional 6.1% of adults had impaired fasting glucose tolerance, increasing to 14.4% for persons aged more than 60 years and with a greater incidence in men than in women [3]. Overall, an estimated 14.4% of the United States population aged more than 20 years and 33.6% of those aged more than 60 years have either diabetes or impaired fasting glucose tolerance. Moreover, type 2 diabetes is now being diagnosed more frequently in children and adolescents concomitant with the increasing prevalence of obesity and

decreased physical activity being seen in this population.

Cardiovascular (CV) diseases are the leading cause of morbidity and mortality in the general population. This baseline risk of CV disease is multiplied two- to fourfold in persons with diabetes mellitus, and the case fatality rate is higher than in nondiabetic patients [4]. CV disease accounts for 65% of deaths in persons with type 2 diabetes mellitus. Much of the morbidity and mortality is from atherosclerotic coronary artery disease, congestive heart failure, and sudden cardiac death. Efforts to reduce the mortality and morbidity related to CV diseases have borne fruit with substantial reduction in CV mortality over the past few decades. Advances in medical therapy and interventional techniques have resulted in only modest improvements in mortality from CV disease in men with diabetes, however, and during the last decade mortality rates of diabetes and CV disease have risen for women (Fig. 1) [5].

The excess CV mortality and morbidity in the diabetic population seems to reflect the strong association of diabetes with insulin resistance and with well-established coronary risk factors. During the past 2 decades, significant advances have been made in elucidating the pathophysiologic determinants and consequences of the metabolic perturbations in the diabetic state. The disease is characterized by insulin resistance and is commonly associated with the metabolic syndrome.

---

* Corresponding author.
*E-mail address:* deed@ucsfresno.edu (P. Deedwania).

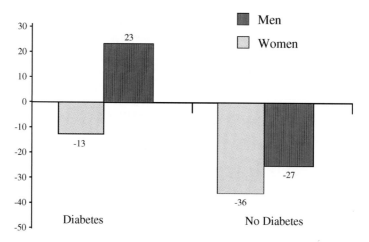

Fig. 1. Change in age-adjusted 8- to 9-year CV mortality in National Health and Nutrition Enhancement Survey over 30 years. (*From* Gu K, Cowie CC, Harris MI. Diabetes and decline in heart disease mortality in US adults. JAMA 1999;281:1291–7; with permission.)

Sensitivity to insulin is variable in the population at large. Cellular insulin resistance develops as the result of a complex interplay of genetic and environmental factors. Hyperinsulinemia occurs as an adaptive response to the increasing insulin resistance. Type 2 diabetes develops when insulin-resistant individuals cannot maintain the degree of excess insulin secretion needed to overcome insulin resistance. There are two aspects to the type 2 diabetic state: hyperglycemia and hyperinsulinemia. Insulin resistance and hyperglycemia seem to set the stage for the development of the metabolic syndrome, characterized by dyslipidemia, hypercoagulability, hypertension, and truncal obesity (Table 1). Several of the metabolic derangements seen with the metabolic syndrome are well-established risk factors for CV disease:

1. Increased fatty acids
2. Increased triglyceride levels
3. Decreased high-density lipoprotein cholesterol (HDL-C)
4. Increased very low density lipoprotein
5. Increased remnant particles
6. Postprandial hyperlipemia
7. Increased small, dense low-density lipoprotein (sdLDL) particles
8. Increased oxidized LDL cholesterol (LDL-C)

Several population-based longitudinal studies have shown that hyperinsulinemia predicts the development of CV disease in individuals without diabetes. Ruige and colleagues [6] performed a meta-analysis of 17 prospective studies, measuring insulin levels in relation to CV outcomes.

They found a statistically significant correlation between insulin levels and the incidence of CV events (relative risk [RR], 1.18; confidence interval, 1.08–1.29). The use of hyperinsulinemia as a surrogate marker for an insulin-resistant state has been confirmed by recent prospective cohort studies showing that insulin resistance, measured by steady-state glucose levels during an insulin suppression test, predicts the risk of CV disease [7,8]. It is unclear whether the insulin resistance per se is directly causative of the increased CV risk. It is, however, well known that metabolic

Table 1
Clinical identification of the metabolic syndrome

| Risk factor | Defining level |
|---|---|
| Abdominal obesity | Waist circumference |
| Men | >40 in (>102 cm) |
| Women | >35 in (>88 cm) |
| Triglycerides | ≥150 mg/dL (≥1.7 mmol/L) |
| High-density lipoprotein cholesterol | |
| Men | <40 mg/dL (<1.04 mmol/L) |
| Women | <50 mg/dL (<1.30 mmol/L) |
| Blood pressure | |
| Systolic | ≥130 mm Hg |
| Diastolic | ≥85 mm Hg |
| Fasting glucose | >100 mg/dL (>5.56 mmol/L) |

Diagnosis is made when ≥3 risk factors are present.
*Modified from* The third report of the Expert Panel on Detection, Evaluation and Treatment of High Blood Cholesterol in Adults (Adult Treatment Panel III). Bethesda (MD): National Institutes of Health; 2002. NIH Publication 02-5215.

abnormalities associated with insulin resistance are established risk factors for CV disease.

The metabolic abnormalities seen with the insulin resistant state seem to antedate the development of overt type 2 diabetes by years. Type 2 diabetes can perhaps be seen as one of the manifestations of the insulin-resistant state. This topic is elegantly covered in another article in this issue, but a brief review is appropriate here. The metabolic syndrome, also known as the insulin resistance syndrome or CV dysmetabolic syndrome, is a constellation of metabolic abnormalities that are associated with a higher risk of CV disease and mortality [9]. The syndrome is a concurrence of three or more of the following abnormalities in an individual:

Waist circumference greater than 102 cm (40 in) in men and 88 cm (35 in) in women
Serum triglyceride level of 150 mg/dL or higher
HDL-C level less than 40 mg/dL in men and 50 mg/dL in women
Blood pressure of 130/85 mm Hg or higher
Fasting glucose level of 110 mg/dL or higher

The metabolic risk factors for CV disease that make up the metabolic syndrome do not directly cause type 2 diabetes but are frequently associated with it. The components of the metabolic syndrome identify individuals at increased risk for CV disease and define various parameters that can be modified to reduce the risk of CV disease. The comprehensive approach to treatment of the diabetic patient should prioritize the goal of reducing CV morbidity and mortality while addressing microvascular complications (nephropathy and retinopathy). Interventions should be targeted at the basic pathophysiologic processes that have been identified as risk factors leading to atherosclerosis and CV disease and are manifest more aggressively in the diabetic patient. The following sections briefly review current literature pertaining to interventions aimed at individual risk factors in the diabetic patient. Subsequently the authors develop the rationale for a comprehensive risk-reduction strategy based on currently available data and explore future directions.

## Significance and treatment of individual risk factors

### Dyslipidemia

Hypertriglyceridemia was one of the first metabolic abnormalities recognized as associated with insulin resistance. The mechanism of the hypertriglyceridemia is understood to result from varying sensitivities to insulin in the tissues in the individual's body. Defects in the ability of insulin to mediate muscle use of glucose and to inhibit lipolysis in adipose tissues seem to be the primary abnormalities causing the insulin-resistant state [10]. The resistance at the level of the muscle and adipose tissue leads to persistently higher ambient levels of insulin and free fatty acids. In response to the higher levels of free fatty acid, the hepatic tissue increases the rate of conversion of free fatty acids to triglycerides. This increased conversion is accentuated by the normal insulin sensitivity of the hepatic tissues in the face of compensatory hyperinsulinemia. The appreciation of the differences in the insulin sensitivity of the various tissues has led to better understanding of the abnormalities caused by insulin resistance. Although the classical diabetic dyslipidemia is characterized by high serum triglyceride levels, low levels of HDL-C, and an increased number of small, dense LDL particles, there are additional lipid abnormalities as well [11,12]. LDL-C is the major cholesterol-rich lipoprotein that mediates the link between serum cholesterol and atherosclerosis. The interaction of LDL-C with monocytes transforms them into the foam cells that are seen in atherosclerotic plaques. This interaction of the monocytes with LDL occurs only when the LDL is modified by acetylation, oxidation, or glycosylation, as realized in diabetes mellitus. Moreover the small, dense LDL particles that are abundant in diabetes mellitus are particularly atherogenic [13]. Thus quantitative and qualitative lipid abnormalities mediate the increased risk of atherosclerosis in diabetes mellitus as shown by the Multiple Risk Factor Intervention Trial Study [14] and the United Kingdom Prospective Diabetes Study (UKPDS) [15]. This topic is discussed more fully elsewhere in this issue.

Dyslipidemia associated with the metabolic syndrome is characterized by increased conversion of HDL-C from large, buoyant $HDL_2$-C particles to more dense $HDL_3$-C particles and conversion of large, buoyant LDL-C particles to small, dense LDL particles. A decrease in plasma levels of cardioprotective $HDL_2$-C accompanied by increase in atherogenic small, dense LDL is associated with a higher risk of coronary artery disease. Stratification of risk factors for coronary artery disease in type 2 diabetes shows that LDL-C and HDL-C levels are the best predictors of coronary heart disease (Table 2). In the diabetic population,

Table 2
Stepwise selection of risk factors* in 2693 diabetics with
dependent variable as time to first event

| Position in model | Variable | P value |
|---|---|---|
| Coronary Artery Disease (n = 280) | | |
| First | LDL cholesterol | <0.0001 |
| Second | HDL cholesterol | 0.0001 |
| Third | Hemoglobin $A_{1c}$ | 0.0022 |
| Fourth | Systolic blood pressure | 0.0065 |
| Fifth | Smoking | 0.056 |

* Adjusted for age and sex.
  *Data from* Turner RC, Millns H, Neil HA, et al. Risk
factors for coronary artery disease in non-insulin
dependent diabetes mellitus: United Kingdom Prospective Diabetes Study (UKPDS: 23). BMJ 1998;316:823–8.

hypertriglyceridemia and low HCL-C levels are
approximately twice as prevalent as in the nondiabetic population, but the prevalence of a high
LDL-C level is similar in the two groups [16].
Although there are no major clinical outcome trials
involving only diabetics, many of the major clinical
intervention trials on dyslipidemia, including the
Scandinavian Simvastatin Survival Study (4S) and
Cholesterol and Recurrent Events (CARE) trials,
have enrolled a substantial number of subjects with
diabetes mellitus [17,18]. In the 4S study, simvastatin led to a 35% decrease in LDL-C resulting in
a 42% decrease in incidence of nonfatal myocardial infarctions and CV mortality. A meta-analysis
of the CARE and Long-term Intervention with
Pravastatin in Ischemic Disease (LIPID) studies
showed a 25% decrease in the incidence of major
coronary events and revascularizations in the subgroup of diabetic patients. Although these studies
included only diabetic patients with established
coronary heart disease, the recently reported findings from the Heart Protection Study support the
use of lipid-lowering therapy in diabetics without
clinically evident atherosclerotic disease [19]. This
study which included almost 4000 diabetics without prior coronary heart disease, demonstrated
a 26% risk reduction of nonfatal myocardial
infarction, death from CV disease, stroke, or revascularizations in the group of subjects treated
with simvastatin. The Heart Protection Study also
challenges the cut point set forth by the Adult
Treatment Panel III (ATP III) of the National
Cholesterol Education Program for target
LDL-C. Trials are being conducted to determine
the desired threshold for LDL-C in secondary
prevention.

More recently, in June 2003, the Collaborative
Atorvastatin Diabetes Study (CARDS), involving
2800 patients with type 2 diabetes, was halted 2
years early because patients allocated to atorvastatin had significant reduction in myocardial
infarction, stroke, and surgical procedures compared with those receiving placebo (Fig. 2) [20].

In this study, 2838 persons with type 2 diabetes
between the ages of 40 and 75 years with no previous history of coronary heart disease, stroke, or
other major CV events and a documented history
of at least one risk factor (retinopathy, micro- or
macroalbuminuria, hypertension, current smoking, LDL levels of 4.14 mmol/L [160 mg/dL] or
lower, and triglyceride levels of 6.78 mmol/L
[600 mg/dL] or lower) were randomly assigned
to either placebo or atrovastatin (10 mg/d).
Patients who received 10 mg of atorvastatin per
day had a 37% reduction in major CV events such
as acute myocardial infarction, stroke, angina,
and revascularization compared with control
patients. In all, 48% fewer patients in the atorvastatin group than in the placebo group suffered
strokes, and all-cause mortality was 27% lower
among patients in the active treatment group
compared with the control group. This landmark
trial was designed specifically to determine the
value of primary prevention of micro- and macrovascular disease in the diabetic population. Treatment with atorvastatin resulted in benefit even in
individuals with LDL levels lower than 100 mg/dL
before treatment.

Hence a wealth of evidence supports the use of
statins for reducing CV risk in diabetics. There
is less evidence for interventions directed at the
diabetic dyslipidemia (high triglyceride and low
HDL levels). In the Veterans Affairs HDL-
cholesterol Intervention Trial (VA-HIT), subjects
received gemfibrozil to increase HDL-C in patients with coronary heart disease and low LDL-C
[21]. In the diabetic subgroup, a 32% decrease in
the incidence of the primary endpoint (combination of nonfatal myocardial infarction, stroke,
and CV death) was noted.

Details of treatment of hyperlipidemia have
been elaborated in another article in this issue. To
summarize, the choice of a particular agent
depends on the baseline lipid profile. A statin
would be the drug of choice if LDL-C is greater
than 100 mg/dL. If the predominant lipid abnormality is hypertriglyceridemia, fibric acid derivative would be the appropriate medicine to use. If
LDL-C is concurrently high, however, treatment
with a statin is necessary. The insulin sensitizers

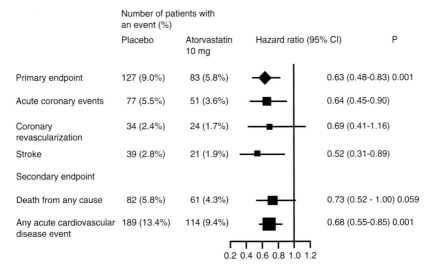

Fig. 2. Effect of treatment on primary and secondary endpoints. (*Adapted from* Colhoun HM, Betteridge DJ, Durrington PN, et al, CARDS investigators. Primary prevention of cardiovascular disease with atorvastatin in type 2 diabetes in the Collaborative Atorvastatin Diabetes Study (CARDS): multicenter randomized placebo-controlled trial. Lancet 2004;364(9435):685–96; with permission.)

(thiazolidinediones, TZDs), have also been shown to have favorable effects on serum triglyceride and HDL-C levels independent of glucose control, and these agents may also reduce the levels of small, dense LDL cholesterol. More long term studies are needed to document the benefits of these agents.

The goals of therapy as recommended by the ATP III of the National Cholesterol Education Program include a LDL-C target of less than 100 mg/dL, a serum triglyceride level less than 150 mg/dL, and an HDL-C level greater than 40 mg/dL [22]. The panel also recommends a secondary target of therapy in non–HDL-C (total cholesterol minus HDL-C). In diabetic individuals with a triglyceride level greater than or equal to 200 mg/dL, the non–HDL-C goal is 130 mg/dL. Although there is no official modification by the National Cholesterol Education Program (NCEP), a recent advisory from the NCEP suggests that because of the associated high risk of coronary events the appropriate LDL target for the diabetic population may be 70 mg/dL [23].

*Hypertension*

Hypertension is seen in about 60% to 80% of individuals with type 2 diabetes. As with the metabolic syndrome, hypertension often predates the manifestation of overt diabetes. There is a significant association between the blood pressure and insulin sensitivity [24,25]. The mechanisms thought to mediate hypertension include insulin resistance and diabetic nephropathy. Insulin resistance and concurrent hyperinsulinemia possibly cause sodium retention by the kidneys, stimulate growth of vascular smooth muscle cell, and affect endothelial function, vascular reactivity, and blood flow.

Several trials have been published regarding the treatment of hypertension in diabetes mellitus. They have shown beyond reasonable doubt that adequate control of blood pressure can protect against macrovascular and microvascular complications. In the Hypertension in Diabetes Study (substudy of the UKPDS), diabetic subjects were randomly assigned into groups with different blood pressure control targets (Fig. 3). After a mean follow-up of more than 8 years, diabetes-related mortality decreased by 32%, incidence of stroke decreased by 44%, and the incidence of congestive heart failure decreased by 56% in the aggressively treated group (mean blood pressure of 144/82 mm Hg during treatment) as compared with the less aggressively treated group (mean blood pressure of 154/87 mm Hg) [26].

In the Hypertension Optimal Treatment (HOT) trial, targeting of diastolic blood pressure to less than 80 mm Hg in diabetic patients was associated with 51% reduction of CV mortality

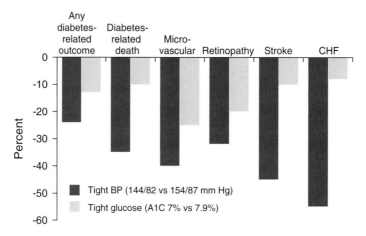

Fig. 3. UKPDS: Comparison between tight control of blood pressure and glycemia on risk of diabetes complications. (*Adapted from* United Kingdom Prospective Diabetes Study Group. Tight blood pressure control and risk of macrovascular and microvascular complications of type 2 diabetes: UKPDS 38. BMJ 1998;317:703–13 and United Kingdom Prospective Diabetes Study Group. Intensive blood-glucose control with sulphonylureas or insulin compared with conventional treatment and risk of complications in patients with type 2 diabetes (UKPDS 33). Lancet 1998;352:837–53; with permission.)

over a 4-year period compared with the group with a target diastolic blood pressure of less than 90 mm Hg [27]. If the diabetic subgroup was removed from the analysis, the benefit in the rest of the population did not achieve statistical significance. Similar data substantiating the benefit of aggressive blood pressure reduction in diabetic patients have been shown in a number of other randomized, controlled trials and are discussed in detail in another article in this issue.

Because of the current evidence from randomized clinical trials, the Joint National Committee on Prevention, Detection, Evaluation and Treatment of High Blood Pressure (in its seventh report, JNC 7) and all other major organizations have recommended a target blood pressure of less than 130/80 mm Hg in patients with diabetes. In patients with diabetic nephropathy and overt proteinuria, the target is 125/75 mm Hg or less [28]. These trials have also shown that adequate control of blood pressure generally requires the use of two or more antihypertensive agents (Fig. 4) [29].

Information regarding the choice of specific antihypertensive agents is more elusive, because most of the trials addressed composite endpoints and not specifically cardioprotection. In general, the degree of blood pressure reduction obtained is more important than the particular agents used, but some conclusions can be drawn from the

available data to help in the choice of antihypertensives. Angiotensin-converting enzyme (ACE) inhibitors have been generally recommended as preferred initial drugs. Persuasive data from the Heart Outcomes Prevention Evaluation (HOPE) study supports of the use of ACE inhibitors [30]. Participants in this study were randomly assigned to either placebo or ramipril. Approximately 3500 diabetic patients with at least one additional classic CV risk factor were enrolled into this trial. Patients with proteinuria, congestive heart failure, recent myocardial infarction, or stroke were excluded, because these conditions are established indications for ACE inhibitors. The combined outcome of myocardial infarction, stroke, and CV deaths was significantly lower in the ramipril-treated group. There was no difference in the blood pressure control between the two groups, and the benefit from ramipril was independent of a patient history of hypertension, CV events, or microalbuminuria.

Some recent studies, however, have shown that angiotensin receptor blockers (ARBs) may be the appropriate initial medication in patients with type 2 diabetes mellitus. For patients with type 1 diabetes and nephropathy, ACE inhibitors remain the cornerstone of therapy. The Reduction of End Points in Non-Insulin-Dependent Diabetes Mellitus with the Angiotensin II Antagonist Losartan (RENAAL) study showed that losartan

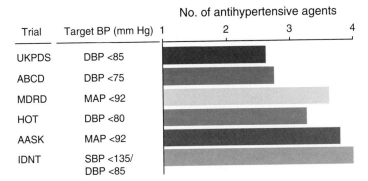

Fig. 4. Multiple antihypertensive agents are needed to achieve target blood pressure. BP, blood pressure; DBP, diastolic blood pressure; MAP, mean arterial pressure; SBP, systolic blood pressure. (*Adapted from* Bakris GL, Williams M, Dworkin L, et al. Preserving renal function in adults with hypertension and diabetes: a consensus approach. Am J Kidney Dis 2000;36(3):646–61; with permission.)

improves renal outcomes in patients with type 2 diabetes and nephropathy over and above the improvement attributable to blood pressure control alone. The renoprotective effect of losartan corresponded to an average delay of 2 years in the need for dialysis or kidney transplantation. The recent RENAAL study and the Irbesartan Type 2 Diabetic Nephropathy Trial found ARBs to offer the greatest benefit for slowing progression of renal disease in type 2 diabetic nephropathy. In contrast, however, the HOPE trial showed that ACE inhibitors, specifically ramipril, have the greatest evidence for prevention of CV outcomes in patients with renal insufficiency, regardless of diabetic status. CV outcomes were secondary endpoints in the RENAAL and IDNT trials, and with the exception of heart failure for losartan, no benefits on CV outcomes were statistically significant. Because evidence has shown that patients with elevated serum creatinine levels ($\geq 1.4$ mg/dL) are just as likely to die from CV disease as to reach end-stage renal disease, it is unclear as to which should be the focus for treatment for clinicians. This question can only be answered by another large, long, randomized, controlled trial using a strictly evidence-based approach. Given the similarity of actions between the ARB and ACE inhibitors, it is likely there is considerable overlap of both benefits and side effects between the two, although ARB may have a lower incidence of cough and hyperkalemia. Trials comparing ARBs with ACE inhibitors are lacking, and more data are needed. Until that information is available, the selection of the appropriate antihypertensive agent should be tailored to the needs of the patient with careful consideration of both

medical and economic factors. Regardless of the choice between an ACE inhibitor and an ARB, however, post hoc analysis of clinical trials and observational data clearly indicate that patients with chronic kidney disease, even if the disease is considered mild (ie, serum creatinine levels $\geq 1.4$ mg/dL), are at significantly greater risk of CV morbidity and mortality than those with better kidney function. Currently, ARBs are the only evidence-based treatment strategy for patients with type 2 diabetes mellitus and proteinuria and are recommended as initial treatment of choice by the National Kidney Foundation [31].

The Losartan Intervention for Endpoint Reduction in Hypertension trial also demonstrated beneficial effects of ARBs in the prevention of stroke events. To conclude, pharmacologic therapy to block the renin-angiotensin system should be mandatory in patients with diabetic nephropathy (including patients with microalbuminuria).

Beta-blockers are recommended for patients with established CV disease, particularly in the presence of coronary artery disease or prior history of myocardial infarction. Findings from the Antihypertensive and Lipid-Lowering Treatment to Prevent Heart Attack Trial suggest that alpha-blockers may have less benefit and could even be harmful when compared with diuretics, amlodipine, or lisinopril [32]. Individuals who have supine hypertension along with significant orthostasis can possibly be treated with short-acting antihypertensive agents such as captopril or oral clonidine at bedtime.

The reduction of elevated blood pressure to the target blood pressure should be the primary goal. This point is well demonstrated in the United

Kingdom Prospective Diabetes Study, which showed no difference in endpoints in patients in whom aggressive blood pressure control was achieved with either captopril or atenolol, whereas a significant difference was noted between the aggressively treated group and the control group. It may be appropriate to select a specific group of antihypertensives for initial treatment because of Specific comorbidities in an individual patient. Also, because most diabetic hypertensive patients require more than two antihypertensive agents, it is prudent to start therapy with at least two drugs, usually as a combination product, to achieve the target blood pressure promptly and to reduce the risk of CV events.

*Hyperglycemia*

A causal relationship between hyperglycemia and microvascular disease is well established. Studies have also documented that glycemic control delays or prevents the manifestations of microvascular disease. The relationship between hyperglycemia and macrovascular disease has been a subject of constant debate, however. The largest study addressing this issue, the UKPDS, was designed to show whether intensive control of glucose lowers the risk of complications compared with conventional treatment in newly diagnosed type 2 diabetics [33,34]. Approximately 2500 patients were enrolled in each group. During a mean follow-up of 10 years, with intensive therapy there was a 12% reduction in any diabetes-related endpoint and a significant reduction in the microvascular endpoints (25% reduction; $P = 0.0099$). A 16% reduction in myocardial infarction ($P = 0.052$) and nonsignificant reductions in diabetes-related and all-cause mortality were noted in the intensively treated group. Thus, although the value of tight glycemic control for prevention of microvascular disease is undisputable, the UKPDS does not strongly suggest a similar benefit in controlling macrovascular disease.

A more recent epidemiologic study, the European Prospective Investigation of Cancer and Nutrition-Norfolk study, found a continuous relationship between all-cause mortality and glycosylated hemoglobin even for values in the nondiabetic range [35]. In this European study, 4662 men aged 45 to 79 years whose glycosylated hemoglobin had been measured at a baseline survey conducted between 1995 and 1997 were followed until December 1999. The main outcome measured was mortality from all causes, from CV disease, from ischemic heart disease, and from other causes. Men with known diabetes had increased mortality from all causes, CV disease, and ischemic disease (RRs, 2.2, 3.3, and 4.2, respectively; $P < 0.001$ independent of age and other risk factors) compared with men without known diabetes. The increased risk of death among men with diabetes was largely explained by the hemoglobin $A_{1c}$ ($HbA_{1c}$) concentration. $HbA_{1c}$ was related to subsequent all-cause, CV, and ischemic heart disease mortality throughout the study population; the lowest rates were seen in those with $HbA_{1c}$ concentrations below 5%. An increase of 1% in $HbA_{1c}$ was associated with a 28% ($P < 0.002$) increase in risk of death independent of age, blood pressure, serum cholesterol, body mass index, and cigarette smoking. This effect remained (RR, 1.46; $P = 0.05$ adjusted for age and risk factors) after men with known diabetes, a $HbA_{1c}$ concentration greater than 7%, or a history of myocardial infarction or stroke were excluded. These data suggest that the 16% risk reduction in the incidence of myocardial infarction found in the UKPDS is a significant difference.

Postprandial hyperglycemia has recently been identified as a potential risk factor for CV disease (Fig. 5) [36]. The study was undertaken by the European Diabetes Epidemiology Study Group in 1997. Baseline data were collected on glucose concentrations at fasting and 2 hours after the 75-g oral glucose tolerance test from 13 prospective European cohort studies, which included 18,048 men and 7316 women aged 30 years or older. Mean follow-up was 7.3 years. The risk of death for the different diagnostic glucose categories was assessed. Within each fasting glucose classification, mortality increased with increasing 2-hour glucose levels. There was, however, no trend for increasing fasting glucose concentrations, for 2-hour glucose classifications of impaired glucose tolerance, or diabetes. This finding suggests that fasting glucose concentrations alone do not identify individuals at increased risk of death associated with hyperglycemia. There are, however, no universally accepted guidelines for therapy. The American College of Endocrinology recommends a 2-hour postprandial target glucose level of less than 140 mg/dL. To summarize, although it remains to be unequivocally proven that intensive glycemic control improves risk of CV outcomes, such control does significantly impact the incidence of microvascular

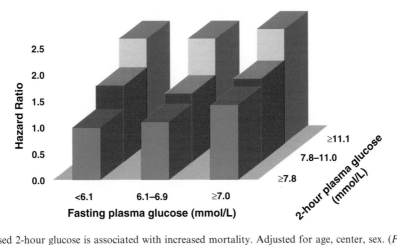

Fig. 5. Increased 2-hour glucose is associated with increased mortality. Adjusted for age, center, sex. (*From* European Diabetes Epidemiology (DECODE) Group. Is the current definition for diabetes relevant to mortality risk from all causes and cardiovascular and noncardiovascular diseases? Diabetes Care 2003;26(3):688–96; with permission.)

complications. Currently, the American Diabetes Association (ADA) recommends a glycosylated hemoglobin goal of 7%, whereas the American College of Endocrinology recommends a goal of less than 6.5%.

The choice of hypoglycemic therapy (as discussed in detail in another article in this issue) should be influenced by consideration of multiple factors including body mass index, renal function, comorbidities, financial issues, and patient preferences. In general, in the absence of contraindications, overweight individuals should initially be treated with metformin. The TZDs, an important therapeutic drug class, are effective in reducing blood sugar. Their hypoglycemic action is mediated by increasing muscle uptake of glucose, thereby decreasing insulin resistance. They also reduce hepatic glucose production. The primary action of these drugs is mediated through activation of the peroxisome proliferator-activated receptor-γ receptor, a nuclear receptor with a regulatory role in differentiation of cells. This receptor is expressed in adipocytes, vascular tissue, and other cell types. These drugs improve endothelial function, reduce intra-abdominal adipose tissue, improve pancreatic beta-cell function, and exert anti-inflammatory actions that may contribute to antiatherosclerotic effects. Ongoing trials are evaluating the nonglycemic effects of these agents on CV outcomes. The prospective pioglitazone clinical trial (PROACTIVE) has randomly assigned more than 5000 patients with type 2 diabetes and documented CV disease to pioglitazone or placebo as add-on therapy to

other hypoglycemic treatment. The Cardiac Outcomes and Regulation of Glycemia in Diabetes (RECORD) study is using rosiglitazone in a similar design. Clinicians should consider using appropriate strategy based on individual patient characteristics and prevailing practices until results of these studies substantiate the benefit of the TZDs in reducing CV disease outcomes.

*Increased thrombotic tendency*

Many prothrombotic factors in the diabetic patient increase the risk for arterial thrombosis leading to myocardial infarction or strokes. These factors include platelet dysfunction (Box 1), increased fibrinogen levels, increased von Willebrand's factor, increased factor VII, increased

---

**Box 1. Platelet dysfunction in diabetes**

1. Reduced membrane fluidity
2. Increased expression of activation-dependent adhesion molecules (eg, P-selectin, GpIIb-IIIa)
3. Increased arachidonic acid metabolism
4. Increased thromboxane A2 synthesis
5. Decreased antioxidant levels
6. Decreased prostacyclin production
7. Decreased nitric oxide production
8. Altered calcium and magnesium homeostasis

plasminogen activator inhibitor type-I, and reduced tissue plasminogen activator levels.

The details of these various coagulation pathway abnormalities have been extensively covered in a recent paper by Sobel [54]. The authors of this article believe it is important to emphasize the role of platelet dysfunction in the setting of diabetes mellitus with a view toward practical implications of antiplatelet therapy.

Multiple biochemical and functional abnormalities in the platelet function have been documented in type 1 and type 2 diabetes and are noted in Box 1. Together these abnormalities lead to increased platelet aggregability and adhesiveness. The correction of this increased platelet aggregability and adhesiveness with antiplatelet agents such as aspirin should logically reduce CV events in diabetics. Although there are no prospective studies designed for investigating the therapeutic role of aspirin in the diabetic cohort, several lines of evidence support its use in reducing CV risk in diabetic patients. In the recently completed Primary Prevention Project study, efficacy of low-dose aspirin (100 mg/d) in primary prevention of CV events was studied in individuals with one or more of the following risk factors: hypertension, hypercholesterolemia, diabetes, obesity, family history of premature myocardial infarction, or advanced age. After a mean follow-up of 3.6 years, there was significantly lower frequency of mortality from CV and of total CV events in the group treated with aspirin [37]. The United States Physicians' Health Study was a 5-year primary prevention trial in nearly 23,000 healthy men that included 533 men with diabetes. Among the diabetic men, 4% of those treated with aspirin (325 mg every other day) had a myocardial infarction, versus 10.1% of those who received placebo (RR, 0.39).

Based on the data from these studies and other collaborative trial data, the ADA recommends the use of enteric-coated aspirin as a primary prevention strategy in patients with diabetes who are classified as high risk [38]. The American Heart Association issued similar recommendations recently, with a dose of 75 to 160 mg/d as primary prevention strategy in individuals with a 10-year coronary heart disease risk of more than 10% [39]. The indications for aspirin use for primary prevention in high-risk diabetic patients are

Obesity
Hypertension
Cigarette smoking
Family history of coronary heart disease
Micro- or microalbuminuria
Atherogenic dyslipidemia

The efficacy of aspirin for secondary prevention of CV events is suggested by a meta-analysis of secondary prevention trials by the Antithrombotic Trialists' Collaboration (ATC). The ATC meta-analysis included 287 trials with total involvement of 212,000 high-risk patients [40]. In more than 4500 patients with diabetes, the incidence of vascular events was reduced from 23.5% with control treatment to 19.3% with antiplatelet therapy ($P < 0.01$). Although the overall incidence of vascular events in the diabetic subgroup was much higher than in the nondiabetic group, the benefit of antiplatelet therapy was comparable in the diabetic and nondiabetic patients. In the HOT study, half of the 1501 patients with diabetes mellitus included in each target group were randomly allocated to receive aspirin. CV events were reduced by 15%, and myocardial infarctions were reduced by 36% compared with placebo. The relative effects of aspirin were similar in nondiabetic and diabetic subjects [27].

Ticlopidine and clopidogrel are thienopyridine antiplatelet agents that inhibit the binding of ADP to the platelet type 2 purinergic receptor, preventing the activation of the GpIIb-IIIa receptor and the subsequent binding of fibrinogen. Thus these agents prevent platelet aggregation. An analysis of the diabetic subgroup in the Clopidogral versus Asprin in Patients at Risk of Ischemic Events study was recently reported [41]. Of 1914 diabetic patients randomly assigned to clopidogrel, 15.6% had the composite vascular primary endpoint, versus 17.7% of 1952 diabetic patients randomly assigned to aspirin therapy ($P = 0.042$). Thus clopidogrel is an effective antiplatelet agent for secondary prevention in diabetic patients, although it is much more expensive than aspirin. Future prospective studies are needed to examine the relative benefits of treatment with clopidogrel versus aspirin in diabetic patients.

## Comprehensive cardiovascular risk reduction in diabetes mellitus

### Multiple risk factor intervention

Although in the past the treatment of diabetes has focused on glycemic control, there is emerging evidence that therapy addressing the concurrent CV risk factors that frequently coexist in the diabetic patient is essential to provide comprehensive CV risk reduction. This approach has

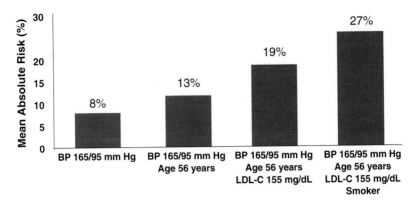

Fig. 6. Multiple risk factors: additive risk. The total severity of multiple low-level risks often exceeds that of a single severely elevated risk. (*From* Grundy SM, Pasternak R, Greenland P, et al. AHA/ACC scientific statement: Assessment of cardiovascular risk by use of multiple-risk-facfor assessment equations: a statement for healthcare professionals from the American Heart Association and the American College of Cardiology. J Am Coll Cardiol 1999;34:1348–59; with permission.)

been strengthened by results from a number of randomized, controlled trials of intensive glycemic control that have failed to show a definite independent link between glycemic control and CV risk reduction. Because the risk of CV events is additive for various risk factors that are frequently present in diabetic patients (Fig. 6), treatment should address all of the CV risk factors in diabetic patients and should not be confined to glycemic control.

Interventions addressing individual CV risk factors in diabetic patients can result in a 15%

to 30% reduction in CV risk. The current stringent treatment targets for glycemic control, blood pressure, and lipid levels have been established as the result of these studies (Table 3).

Although addressing individual risk factors in the diabetic patient is a logical extension of the findings from currently available evidence, this approach has limited potential in achieving the maximal attainable benefit from reduction of CV risk. A more appropriate approach would be to address multiple risk factors concurrently with the hope of obtaining a comprehensive reduction in

Table 3
Goals for risk factor management in diabetes

| Risk factor | Goal of therapy | Reference |
|---|---|---|
| Cigarette smoking | Complete cessation | 47 |
| Blood pressure | <130/80 mm Hg | 46,47 |
| (with proteinuria) | <125/75 | 46,47 |
| LDL cholesterol | <100 mg/dL | 47,52 |
| | <70 mg/dL in high risk[a] | |
| Triglycerides 200–499 mg/dL | Non-HDL cholesterol < 130 mg/dL | 52 |
| HDL cholesterol <40 mg/dL | Raise HDL | 52 |
| Prothrombotic state | Low-dose aspirin therapy (patients with congestive heart disease and other high-risk patients) | 47 |
| Glucose | Hemoglobin $A_{1C}$ < 7% | 47 |
| Overweight and obesity (body mass index ≥25 kg/m$^2$) | Lose 10% of body weight in 1 year | 28 |
| Physical inactivity | Exercise prescription dependent on patient status | 47 |
| Adverse nutrition | Diets low in saturated fat and lower glycemic index (when necessary with caloric concentration) | 47,53,28,52,51 |

[a] Per recent advisory from NCEP.

risk. Although such a strategy would require considerable effort on the part of the physician and the patient, available data suggest that the approach of comprehensive risk reduction is beneficial in the management of the diabetic patient.

The Steno-2 Trial prospectively examined the benefits of multifactorial intervention in reducing CV disease in 160 patients with microalbuminuria [42]. One hundred sixty patients with type 2 diabetes and microalbuminuria were randomly assigned to receive either conventional care or intensive treatment. Eighty patients were randomly assigned to receive conventional treatment for multiple risk factors from their general practitioner, following the 1998 recommendations of the Danish Medical Association that were revised in 2000. The remaining 80 patients were randomly assigned to undergo intensive multifactorial intervention with strict treatment goals (Table 4) to be achieved through behavior modification and a stepwise introduction of pharmacologic therapy overseen by a project team consisting of a physician, nurse, and dietician. Therapy was intended to maintain glycosylated hemoglobin values below 6.5%, blood pressure below 130/80 mm Hg, cholesterol levels below 175 mg/dL, and triglyceride levels below 150 mg/dL. Intensive therapy involved clinic visits with the multidisciplinary diabetes team every 3 months. During these visits, patients received advice regarding lifestyle adjustment (eg, diet, exercise, smoking cessation courses), and medications were adjusted to achieve treatment targets for hypertension,

dyslipidemia, microalbuminuria, and hyperglycemia along with aspirin for secondary prevention of CV disease. Dietary intervention was aimed at a total fat intake of less than 30% of daily energy intake and an intake of saturated fatty acids representing less than 10% of the daily energy intake. Light to moderate exercise for at least 30 minutes three to five times a week was recommended, and all smoking patients and their spouses were invited to participate in smoking-cessation courses. All patients were prescribed an ACE inhibitor in a dose equivalent to 50 mg of captopril two times/d or, if the ACE-inhibitor was contraindicated, an ARB in a dose equivalent to 50 mg of losartan two times/d, irrespective of blood pressure. After 2000, these medications were also routinely prescribed for patients in the conventional-therapy group (Table 5).

The primary endpoint of this open, parallel trial was a composite of death from CV causes, nonfatal myocardial infarction, nonfatal stroke, revascularization, and amputation. After a mean follow-up period of 7.8 years, the declines in glycosylated hemoglobin values, systolic and diastolic blood pressure, serum cholesterol and triglyceride levels, and urinary albumin excretion rate were all significantly greater in the intensive-therapy group than in the conventional-therapy group. There was also significant reduction of CV disease, nephropathy, retinopathy, and autonomic neuropathy. The groups did not differ significantly in the number of patients who reported at least one minor episode of

Table 4

Treatment goals for the conventional therapy group and the intensive therapy group

| Variable | Conventional therapy | | Intensive therapy | |
|---|---|---|---|---|
| | 1993–1999 | 2000–2001 | 1993–1999 | 2000–2001 |
| Systolic blood pressure (mm Hg) | <160 | <135 | <140 | <130 |
| Diastolic blood pressure (mm Hg) | <95 | <85 | <85 | <80 |
| Glycosylated hemoglobin (%) | <7.5 | <6.5 | <6.5 | <6.5 |
| Fasting serum total cholesterol (mg/dL)[a] | <250 | <190 | <190 | <175 |
| Fasting serum triglycerides (mg/dL)[b] | <195 | <180 | <150 | <150 |
| Treatment with ACE-I irrespective of blood pressure | No | Yes | Yes | Yes |
| Aspirin therapy | | | | |
|   For patients with known ischemia | Yes | Yes | Yes | Yes |
|   For patients with peripheral vascular disease | No | No | Yes | Yes |
|   For patients without coronary heart disease or peripheral vascular disease | No | No | No | Yes |

[a] To convert values for cholesterol to millimoles per liter, multiply by 0.02586.

[b] To convert values for triglycerides to millimoles per liter, multiply by 0.01129.

*Data from* Gaede P, Vedel P, Larsen N, et al. Multifactorial intervention and cardiovascular disease in patients with type 2 diabetes. N Engl J Med 2003;348:383–93. Copyright © 2003 Massachusetts Medical Society.

Table 5
Treatment in patients with type 2 diabetes and microalbuminuria in Steno-2

| | Start of study period | | End of study period | | |
|---|---|---|---|---|---|
| Variable | Conventional therapy (N = 80) | Intensive therapy (N = 80) | Conventional therapy (N = 63) | Intensive therapy (N = 67) | P value |
| Glucose-lowering treatment | | | | | |
| Diet alone (no. of patients) | 21 | 28 | 4 | 1 | 0.15 |
| Oral hypoglycemic agent (no. of patients) | 48 | 47 | 38 | 50 | 0.14 |
| Insulin (no. of patients) | 11 | 5 | 34 | 38 | 0.91 |
| Both agents (no. of patients) | 1 | 0 | 13 | 22 | 0.14 |
| Insulin dose (IU) | | | | | 0.91 |
| Median | 30 | 42 | 64 | 62 | |
| Range | 14–142 | 10–52 | 12–360 | 12–260 | |
| Antihypertensive treatment (no. of patients) | | | | | |
| ACE-I | 16 | 15 | 32 | 53 | 0.002 |
| Angiotensin II-receptor antagonist | 0 | 0 | 12 | 31 | 0.002 |
| Both | 0 | 0 | 0 | 19 | <0.001 |
| Diuretic | 17 | 22 | 39 | 38 | 0.42 |
| Calcium-channel blocker | 5 | 11 | 18 | 24 | 0.45 |
| Beta-blocker | 8 | 1 | 13 | 10 | 0.35 |
| Other | 1 | 1 | 4 | 3 | 0.61 |
| Any | 33 | 33 | 52 | 66 | 0.009 |
| Lipid-lowering treatment (no. of patients) | | | | | |
| Statin | 0 | 2 | 14 | 57 | <0.001 |
| Fibrate | 1 | 1 | 3 | 1 | 0.27 |
| Both | 0 | 0 | 0 | 1 | 1.00 |
| Aspirin (no. of patients) | 11 | 10 | 35 | 58 | <0.001 |
| Vitamin-mineral supplement (no. of patients) | 0 | 0 | 0 | 42 | <0.001 |
| Hormone replacement (no. of patients) | 3 | 2 | 2 | 1 | 0.61 |

P values are for the difference between the groups at the end of the study.

Data from Gaede P, Vedel P, Larsen N, et al. Multifactorial intervention and cardiovascular disease in patients with type 2 diabetes. N Engl J Med 2003;348:383–93. Copyright © 2003 Massachusetts Medical Society.

hypoglycemia at the 4- or 8-year examination. The reduction in macrovascular events was 53% in the intensive-treatment group. The benefits of intensive treatment were evident at 1 year in the intensive-treatment group. This study indicates that five patients need to be treated intensively over 7 years to prevent one event (Figs. 7, 8). The treatment targets in the intensively treated group were rather liberal compared with current guidelines (see Table 3). It is conceivable that the reduction of events in the intensively treated group would have been more substantial if treatment targets had been set to current guidelines. Although the results of this study are exciting, more data are needed. Large, randomized, controlled trials in a wide variety of diabetic patients with various risk stratifications are needed to verify and reproduce similar results. Additionally trials need to be conducted using the newer pharmacologic agents, specially the TZDs, which were not used in the Steno-2 trial. Any such trial should also make a concerted effort to attain current recommended treatment goals regarding glycemic control, lipid levels, and blood pressure control. Although data from future trials might be useful in building the evidence base, feasibility could be an issue because current guidelines might make less intensive treatment ethically questionable. The results of ongoing trials such as Action Control CV Risk in Diabetes and Bypass Angioplasty Revascularization Investigation conducted by the National Institutes of Health should provide with useful data in this regard, however.

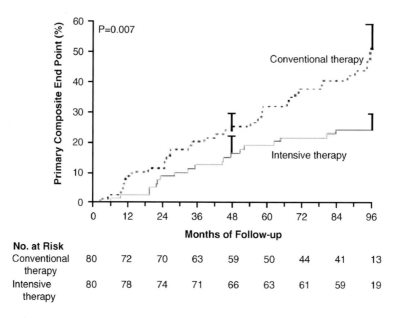

Fig. 7. Kaplan-Meier estimates of the composite endpoint of death from CV causes, nonfatal myocardial infarction, coronary artery bypass grafting, percutaneous coronary intervention, nonfatal stroke, amputation, or surgery for peripheral atherosclerotic artery disease in the conventional therapy group and the intensive therapy group. (*From* Gaede P, Vedel P, Larsen N, et al. Multifactorial intervention and cardiovascular disease in patients with type 2 diabetes. N Engl J Med 2003;348:383–93; with permission. Copyright © 2003 Massachusetts Medical Society.)

## Practical considerations

Implementation of an intensive and multifactorial treatment strategy requires extensive resources including a multidisciplinary team and a greater time commitment per patient. Other factors to consider in the equation are patient characteristics and behaviors that may affect adherence to treatment and cost issues related to multiple medications needed to meet the stringent treatment targets. The cost-effectiveness analysis done by

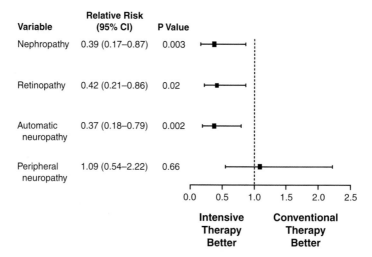

Fig. 8. Relative risk of the development or progression of nephropathy, retinopathy, and autonomic and peripheral neuropathy during the average follow-up of 7.8 years in the intensive therapy group, as compared with the conventional therapy group. (*From* Gaede P, Vedel P, Larsen N, et al. Multifactorial intervention and cardiovascular disease in patients with type 2 diabetes. N Engl J Med 2003;348:383–93; with permission. Copyright © 2003 Massachusetts Medical Society.)

the Diabetes Cost-effectiveness Group of the Centers for Disease Control provides some insights into these issues [43]. A hypothetical cohort of individuals with newly diagnosed type 2 diabetes in the United States was used. A Markov model of type 2 diabetes disease progression was used to calculate incremental cost-effectiveness ratios for the interventions. Interventions considered were sulfonylurea or insulin for intensive glycemic control, ACE inhibitors or beta-blockers for intensified hypertension control, and pravastatin for reducing the serum cholesterol level. Intensified hypertension control was found to reduce costs and improve health outcomes as compared with moderate hypertension control. Although intensive glycemic control and reduction in serum cholesterol level also improved health outcomes, these goals were achieved at increased costs. This analysis raises questions regarding the most appropriate and economically feasible guidelines from the perspective of public health. Although more studies evaluating the cost–benefit analysis of various targeted interventions are certainly needed to determine whether comprehensive risk reduction is the most appropriate and cost-effective strategy in the diabetic patient, the clinician must now rely on the available data and good clinical judgment. The clinician should consider the specific risk profile for the given patient and institute the appropriate risk-reduction strategy to achieve the greatest benefit. For example, in the case of a diabetic patient with microalbuminuria or a strong family history of premature coronary artery disease, the predictable high risk of CV events makes it mandatory to institute aggressive management of all the modifiable risk factors at the earliest possible time.

## Current state of affairs and future directions

Although the wisdom of addressing multiple risk factors seems to be intuitively obvious, this approach is not what transpires in practice. Data from National Health and Nutrition Enhancement Survey 1999–2000 reveal that only 37% of adults with diagnosed diabetes in the United States are achieving the ADA goal of glycosylated hemoglobin levels less than 7% [44]. In addition, 37% of adults with diagnosed diabetes have glycosylated hemoglobin levels greater than 8%. Only 36% of individuals with diabetes have achieved the current goals for blood pressure set in the JNC 7. More than half the individuals with diagnosed diabetes have cholesterol levels above 200 mg/dL. Thus, there is great room for improvement in the provision of diabetes care and education to capitalize on knowledge currently available. A systematic approach to the treatment of diabetes that addresses multiple risk factors is needed. The increased awareness of the importance of controlling risk factors for vascular disease among adults with diabetes has led to national programs such as the NCEP's campaign, "Control of ABCs" (in which "A" stands for $HbA_{1c}$, "B" stands for blood pressure, and "C" stands for cholesterol) and the Diabetes Quality Improvement Project [45,46]. Techniques in comprehensive risk reduction could involve the use of standardized flow charts and diet and exercise protocols that could be developed at various clinic sites to expedite visits and establish a uniform standard of care. Trials are still needed to determine the intervention or combination of interventions that could provide the maximal benefits, the extent of these benefits and the most cost-effective approaches that could be applied to a wide group of patients.

The best approach for the problem of diabetes mellitus and associated CV disease is to prevent or delay the onset of diabetes mellitus. A truly comprehensive approach to reducing the risks posed by diabetes should explore the possibility of preventing or delaying the onset of diabetes. From a public health perspective, this approach, with the potential of wide application, might be the most cost effective strategy. Of course, the assumption is that prevention of diabetes will also lead to prevention of atherosclerosis, and this assumption is yet to be substantiated by prospective trials. To demonstrate this association, individuals at risk must be identified early in the course of development of the disease. For this reason the Western Working Group, NCEP, ADA, and other major groups have emphasized the importance of the metabolic syndrome as a potential prediabetic state [9,22,47]. Although data are lacking regarding the benefit of intervention in patients with the metabolic syndrome, simple measures such as weight reduction and regular activity can reduce the risk of developing diabetes mellitus and potentially reduce CV disease.

During the transition from euglycemia to overt diabetes, many patients go through a phase of impaired glucose tolerance or impaired fasting glucose, defined by an oral glucose tolerance test finding of 140 to 190 mg/dL and a fasting plasma glucose level of 110 to 125 mg/dL, respectively. As discussed in another article in this issue, substantial trial evidence shows that the onset of diabetes can be prevented or at least delayed in this cohort of individuals [48,49]. Emerging evidence suggests that prevention of diabetes can indeed be beneficial in reducing the risk of CV events. In the STOP-NIDDM trial, treatment with acarbose was associated with a 25% risk reduction in development of diabetes and resulted in significant reduction in CV events [50]. The results of the STOP-NIDDM trial are indeed interesting and provocative, but they need to be confirmed by other prospective, randomized clinical trials.

The prevention of diabetes may indeed be attractive, because the interventions needed are generally less expensive and would translate to large reductions in health care expenditure with the potential for reduction of macrovascular disease. Therefore, a comprehensive approach to the risk reduction of CV events associated with diabetes should incorporate diabetes prevention strategies, especially as a public health measure. It is worthwhile to remember the aphorism, "an ounce of prevention is worth a pound of cure."

## Summary

Diabetic patients are at increased risk of CV disease morbidity and mortality. In the past, treatment of diabetic patients largely focused on tight glycemic control. A number of studies, however, have shown that aggressive control of blood pressure and hyperlipidemia and the institution of antithrombotic therapy are beneficial in reducing the risk of CV events in the diabetic patient. Although in general these studies have shown a 15% to 30% reduction in the RR of CV events, the absolute risk of CV events remains high in the intervention group, probably because most of these trials have not incorporated a comprehensive risk-reduction strategy. Emerging data suggest that a therapeutic strategy using appropriate therapy to address multiple components of CV risks in diabetic patients is indeed beneficial in reducing the absolute risk of CV events. Although more data are needed to substantiate the benefits, feasibility, and cost effectiveness of such therapy, there is sufficient evidence for the clinician to provide an individualized approach and to consider aggressive intervention to minimize the predictable risk of CV events in the high-risk diabetic patient.

## References

[1] King H, Aubert RE, Herman WH. Global burden of diabetes, 1995–2025: prevalence, numerical estimates, and projections. Diabetes Care 1998;21: 1414–31.

[2] Centers for Disease Control. National Health and Nutrition Examination Survey 1999–2000 data files. Available at: http://www.cdc.gov/nchs/about/major/nhanes/NHANES99_00.htm. Accessed December 21, 2004.

[3] International Diabetes Federation. IGT/IFG Consensus. Statement Report of an expert consensus workshop, August 1–4, 2001. Stoke Poges, United Kingdom. Impaired glucose tolerance and impaired fasting glycemia: the current status on definition and intervention. Diabet Med 2002;19:708–23.

[4] Saydah SH, Eberhardt MS, Loria CM, et al. Age and the burden of death attributable to diabetes in the United States. Am J Epidemiol 2002;156: 714–9.

[5] Gu K, Cowie CC, Harris MI. Diabetes and decline in heart disease mortality in US adults. JAMA 1999; 281:1291–7.

[6] Ruige JB, Assendelft WJ, Dekker JM, et al. Insulin and risk of CV disease: a meta-analysis. Circulation 1998;97(10):996–1001.

[7] Yip J, Facchini FS, Reaven GM. Resistance to insulin-mediated glucose disposal as a predictor of cardiovascular disease. J Clin Endocrinol Metab 1998;83:2773–6.

[8] Facchini FS, Hua N, Abbasi F, et al. Insulin resistance as a predictor of age related diseases. J Clin Endocrinol Metab 2001;86:3574–8.

[9] Fagan TC, Deedwania PC. The cardiovascular dysmetabolic syndrome. Am J Med 1998;105(1A): 77S–82S.

[10] Abbasi F, McLaughlin T, Lamendola C, et al. The relationship between glucose disposal in response to physiological hyperinsulinemia and basal glucose and free fatty acid concentrations in healthy volunteers. J Clin Endocrinol Metab 2000;85: 1252–4.

[11] Taskinen MR, Smith U. Lipid disorders in NIDDM: implications for treatment. J Intern Med 1998;244: 361–70.

[12] Garg A. Treatment of diabetic dyslipidemia. Am J Cardiol 1998;81:47B–51B.

[13] Veniant MM, Sullivan MA, Kim SK, et al. Defining the atherogenicity of large and small lipoproteins containing apolipoprotein B100. J Clin Invest 2000; 106:1501–10.

[14] Stamler J, Vaccaro I, Neaton JD, et al. Diabetes, other risk factors, and 12-yr cardiovascular mortality for men screened in the Multiple Risk Factor Intervention Trial. Diabetes Care 1993;16: 434–44.

[15] Turner RC, Millns H, Neil HA, et al. Risk factors for coronary artery disease in non-insulin dependent

diabetes mellitus: United Kingdom Prospective Diabetes Study (UKPDS: 23). BMJ 1998;316: 823–8.

[16] Garg A, Grundy SM. Management of dyslipidemia in NIDDM. Diabetes Care 1990;13:153–69.

[17] Pyorola K, Pederson TR, Kjekshus J, et al. Cholesterol lowering with simvastatin improves prognosis of diabetic patients with coronary heart disease: a sub-group analysis of the Scandinavian Simvastatin Survival Study (4S). Diabetes Care 1997;20: 614–20.

[18] Goldberg RB, Mellies MJ, Sacks FM, et al, for the CARE investigators. Cardiovascular events and their reduction with pravastatin in diabetic and glucose- intolerant myocardial infarction survivors with average cholesterol and recurrent events (CARE) trial. Circulation 1998;98:2513–9.

[19] Collins R, Armitage J, Parish S, et al. Heart Protection Study Collaborative Group. MRC/BHF heart protection study of cholesterol-lowering with simvastatin in 5963 people with diabetes: a randomised placebo-controlled trial. Lancet 2003;361(9374): 2005–16.

[20] Colhoun HM, Betteridge DJ, Durrington PN, et al, for the CARDS investigators. Primary prevention of cardiovascular disease with atorvastatin in type 2 diabetes in the Collaborative Atorvastatin Diabetes Study (CARDS): multicenter randomized placebo-controlled trial. Lancet 2004;364(9435): 685–96.

[21] Rubins HB, Robins SJ, Collins D, et al, for the Veterans Affairs High-Density Lipoprotein Cholesterol Intervention Trial Study Group. Gemfibrozil for the secondary prevention of coronary heart disease in men with low levels of high- density lipoprotein cholesterol. N Engl J Med 1999;341:410–8.

[22] Expert Panel on Detection. Evaluation, and Treatment of High Blood Cholesterol in Adults. Executive summary of the third report of the National Cholesterol Education Program (NCEP) Expert Panel on Detection, Evaluation, and Treatment of High Blood Cholesterol in Adults (Adult Treatment Panel III). JAMA 2001;285:2486–97.

[23] Grundy SM, Cleeman JI, Bairey Merz CN, et al, for the Coordinating Committee of the National Cholesterol Education Program. Implications of recent clinical trials for the National Cholesterol Education Program Adult Treatment Panel III guidelines. Circulation 2004;110:227–39.

[24] Ferrannini E, Buzzigoli G, Bonadona R. Insulin resistance in essential hypertension. N Engl J Med 1987;317:350–7.

[25] Swislocki ALM, Hoffman BB, Raven GM. Insulin resistance, glucose intolerance and hyperinsulinemia in patients with hypertension. Am J Hypertens 1989; 2:419–23.

[26] United Kingdom Prospective Diabetes Study Group. Tight blood pressure control and risk of macrovascular and microvascular complications

of type 2 diabetes: UKPDS 38. BMJ 1998;317: 703–13.

[27] Hansson L, Zanchetti A, Carruthers SG, et al. Effects of intensive blood pressure lowering and low-dose aspirin in patients with hypertension: principal results of the hypertension optimal treatment (HOT) randomised trial. Lancet 1998;351: 1755–62.

[28] Wright JT Jr, Jones DW, Green LA, et al. The seventh report of the Joint National Committee on Prevention, Detection, Evaluation and Treatment of High Blood Pressure: the JNC 7 report. JAMA 2003;289:2560–71.

[29] Bakris GL, Williams M, Dworkin L, et al. Preserving renal function in adults with hypertension and diabetes: a consensus approach. Am J Kidney Dis 2000;36(3):646–61.

[30] Heart Outcomes Prevention Evaluation (HOPE) Study Investigators. Effects of ramipril on cardiovascular and microvascular outcomes in people with diabetes mellitus: results of the HOPE Study and MICRO-HOPE substudy. Lancet 2000;355: 253–9 [published correction appears in Lancet 2000;356:850].

[31] Kidney Disease Outcome Quality Initiative. K/DOQI clinical practice guidelines for chronic kidney disease: evaluation, classification, and stratification. Am J Kidney Dis 2002;39(2 Suppl 1):S1–266.

[32] Poulter N, Williams B. Doxazosin for the management of hypertension: implications of the findings of the ALLHAT Trial. Am J Hypertens 2001;14: 1170–2.

[33] United Kingdom Prospective Diabetes Study Group. Intensive blood-glucose control with sulphonylureas or insulin compared with conventional treatment and risk of complications in patients with type 2 diabetes (UKPDS 33). Lancet 1998; 352:837–53.

[34] United Kingdom Prospective Diabetes Study Group. Effect of intensive blood glucose control with metformin on complications in overweight patients with type 2 diabetes (UKPDS 34). Lancet 1998;352:854–65.

[35] Khaw KT, Wareham N, Luben R, et al. Glycated hemoglobin, diabetes, and mortality in men in Norfolk cohort of European prospective investigation of cancer and nutrition (EPIC-Norfolk). BMJ 2001; 322(7277):15–8.

[36] European Diabetes Epidemiology (DECODE) Group. Is the current definition for diabetes relevant to mortality risk from all causes and cardiovascular and noncardiovascular diseases? Diabetes Care 2003;26(3):688–96.

[37] Collaborative Group of the Primary Prevention Project. Low-dose aspirin and vitamin E in people at cardiovascular risk: a randomized trial in general practice. Lancet 2002;357:89–95.

[38] Colwell JA. Aspirin therapy in diabetes. Diabetes Care 2003;26(Suppl 1):S87–8.

[39] United States Preventive Services Task Force. Aspirin for the primary prevention of cardiovascular events: recommendations and rationale. Ann Intern Med 2001;136:157–60.

[40] Antithrombotic Trialists' Collaboration. Collaboration meta-analysis of randomized trials of antiplatelet therapy for prevention of death, myocardial infarction, and stroke in high risk patients. BMJ 2002;324:71–86.

[41] Bhatt D, Marso S, Hirsh A, Ringleb P, et al. Amplified benefit of clopidogrel versus aspirin in patients with diabetes mellitus. Am J Cardiol 2002;90: 625–8.

[42] Gaede P, Vedel P, Larsen N, et al. Multifactorial intervention and cardiovascular disease in patients with type 2 diabetes. N Engl J Med 2003;348: 383–93.

[43] Hoerger TJ, Bethke AD, Richter A, et al. The CDC Diabetes Cost-Effectiveness Group. Cost-effectiveness of intensive glycemic control, intensified hypertension control, and serum cholesterol level reduction for type 2 diabetes. JAMA 2002; 287:2542–51.

[44] Saydah S, Fradkin J, Cowie C. Poor control of risk factors for vascular disease among adults with previously diagnosed diabetes. JAMA 2004;291: 335–42.

[45] Clark CM, Fradkin JE, Hiss RG, et al. The National Diabetes Education Program, changing the way diabetes is treated. Diabetes Care 2001;24:617–8.

[46] Fleming BB, Greenfield S, Engelgau MM, et al. The Diabetes Quality Improvement Project: moving science into health policy to gain an edge on the diabetes epidemic. Diabetes Care 2001;24:1815–20.

[47] American Diabetes Association. Standards of Medical Care in Diabetes—position statements. Diabetes Care 2004;27:S15–35.

[48] Lindstrom J, Eriksson JG, Valle TT, et al. Prevention of diabetes mellitus in subjects with impaired glucose tolerance in the Finnish diabetes prevention study: results from a randomized clinical trial. J Am Soc Nephrol 2003;14(7 Suppl 2):S108–13.

[49] The DPP Research Group. Reduction in the incidence of type 2 diabetes with lifestyle intervention or metformin. N Engl J Med 2002;346: 393–403.

[50] Chiasson JL, Josse RG, Gomis R, et al, for the STOP-NIDDM Trial Research Group. Acarbose for prevention of type 2 diabetes mellitus: the STOP-NIDDM randomised trial. Lancet 2002;359: 2072–7.

[51] Joint National Committee on Detection, Evaluation and Treatment of High Blood Pressure: The seventh report of the Joint National Committee on Detection, Evaluation and Treatment of High Blood Pressure (JNC 7). JAMA 2003;289(19): 2560–72.

[52] Clinical guidelines on the identification, evaluation, and treatment of overweight and obesity in adults: the evidence report published by the National Institutes of Health, National Heart, Lung, and Blood Institute in June 1998.

[53] Lauber RP, Sheard NF. The American Heart Association dietary guidelines for 2000: a summary report. Nutr Rev 2001;59(9):298–306.

[54] Sobel BE, Schneider DJ. Platelet function, coagulopathy and impaired fibrinolysis in diabetes. Cardiol Clin 2004;22(4):511–26.

ELSEVIER
SAUNDERS

Cardiol Clin 23 (2005) 211–220

CARDIOLOGY
CLINICS

# Prevention of Cardiovascular Outcomes in Type 2 Diabetes Mellitus: Trials on the Horizon

John B. Buse, MD, PhD[a],*, Julio Rosenstock, MD[b,c]

[a]Divisions of Endocrinology and General Medicine and Clinical Epidemiology,
Diabetes Care Center, University of North Carolina School of Medicine, CB #7110,
5039 Old Clinic Building, Chapel Hill, NC 27599-7110, USA
[b]Dallas Diabetes and Endocrine Center,
7777 Forest Lane, C-618, Dallas, TX 75230, USA
[c]University of Texas Southwestern Medical School, Dallas, TX, USA

Type 2 diabetes mellitus is a clinical syndrome characterized by hyperglycemia in which early cardiovascular (CV) death is the predominant clinical outcome. In the last 20 years several clinical trials have demonstrated unequivocally techniques that reduce the risk for CV events in patients who have diabetes mellitus; these studies form the basis for current guidelines regarding management of patients who have diabetes mellitus, specifically in the areas of lipid modification, blood pressure reduction, modulation of the renin-angiotensin system, antiplatelet therapy, and invasive revascularization procedures.

Despite the many published clinical trials, reviews, and guidelines on diabetes mellitus and cardiovascular disease (CVD), large untested areas of accepted clinical practice remain. Although interventional trials strongly support the notion that more intensive glycemic control is associated with a reduction in microvascular complications, there is only epidemiologic basis for the causal link between glucose control and CVD. Outcomes from the adequately powered clinical trials addressing the relationship between intervention to lower glucose and CV events are awaited with great interest. Furthermore, no outcomes studies have been conducted with insulin analogs or thiazolidinediones. Clinical practice is informed by the best available data, but epidemiologic studies can lead one astray, as was the case with hormone replacement therapy as a technique to reduce CVD [1].

This article focuses on the continuing clinical trials in patients who have diabetes mellitus and prediabetes in which CVD outcomes—specifically CV death, myocardial infarction (MI), and stroke—are examined as primary outcomes. These trials were identified using three approaches:

1. Searching www.clinicaltrials.gov, a National Institutes of Health (NIH)–funded website that provides "regularly updated information about federally and privately supported clinical research in human volunteers" with almost 200 diabetes mellitus trials posted [2];
2. Hand-searching titles and abstracts for over 3000 citations identified in the National Library of Medicine PubMed System describing clinical trials in diabetes mellitus cited over the prior 5 years; and
3. Querying thought leaders in diabetes mellitus and CVD as well as representatives of the NIH's National Heart Lung and Blood Institute and National Institute on Diabetes, Digestive and Kidney Diseases.

This article was originally published in *Endocrinology and Metabolism Clinics of North America* 34:1, 2005.

Dr. Buse is supported in part by National Institutes of Health Grants RR00046, HC9961, and DK061223.

\* Corresponding author.

*E-mail address:* jbuse@med.unc.edu (J.B. Buse).

This is undoubtedly an incomplete representation of the work being conducted in this regard and the authors recognize in advance the potential intellectual risk of any oversights. Many additional studies examine only intermediate surrogate outcomes (eg, intravascular ultrasound, carotid intimal thickness, and CV risk markers), but unfortunately, there is little published information about them. Various search engines were used to identified design details from study websites and press releases, which are referenced to the extent that they provided additional details.

For purposes of discussion these trials have been grouped based on general themes:

- Trials that examine glycemic targets,
- Trials that examine interventional techniques of glucose lowering, and
- Trials that examine nonglycemic interventions.

Some studies involve designs (eg, factorial designs) in which more than one intervention is examined. In those cases, the theme of the study will be introduced in the earlier section and additional details regarding other interventions in subsequent sections.

## Trials examining glycemic targets

The most hotly debated clinical questions in diabetes mellitus are whether glycemic control is associated with a reduction in CVD outcomes and how low a glycemic target should be pursued. Because the risk for severe hypoglycemia increases as lower targets are achieved, there is a floor below which benefits will be counterbalanced by risk. Guidelines suggest that hemoglobin A1c (HbA1c) targets of less than 7% [3], 6.5% [4], or 6.1% [5] are appropriate. These goals have been

imputed by examining epidemiologic studies because there are no CVD outcomes studies in diabetes mellitus that have provided clear-cut, statistically significant reductions in endpoints. Indeed, no reported interventional outcome study has yet achieved the above recommended A1c targets. The clinical trial that comes closest to meeting such criteria is the United Kingdom Prospective Diabetes Study (UKPDS) [6], which suggests that the method of glucose lowering may be more important than the target or the average level of glycemia achieved [7]. Three current clinical trials are testing directly the hypothesis that glucose lowering in the setting of type 2 diabetes mellitus is associated with a reduction in CVD events (Table 1).

### ADVANCE

In the ADVANCE trial (Action in Diabetes and Vascular Disease: Preterax and Diamicron MR Controlled Evaluation), 11,140 patients who have type 2 diabetes mellitus were recruited in 200 centers in Australia, Asia, Europe, and North America. The eligibility criteria are broad: diagnosis of type 2 diabetes mellitus after 30 years of age, age 55 or more years, and high risk for CVD. Patients are randomized in a $2 \times 2$ factorial design to an open-label, modified-release (MR) sulfonylurea (gliclazide MR)–based intensive treatment with a goal of achieving a HbA1c level of 6.5% or less versus standard care for glycemia as well as a blood pressure intervention (see later discussion). There are two primary endpoints: (1) the composite of stroke, MI, and CV death, and (2) the composite of new or worsening nephropathy or microvascular eye disease. The scheduled postrandomization follow-up is 4.5 years. The study is designed to provide 90% power to detect

Table 1
Studies of glycemic control and its relationship to cardiovascular disease outcomes

| Study [Ref.] | No. of participants | Follow-up, years | A1c target, % | | Expected results |
|---|---|---|---|---|---|
| | | | Intensive | Standard | |
| ADVANCE [8–10] | 11,140 | ~4.5 | ≤ 6.5 | ~7.5 (usual care) | 2006 |
| VADT [11] | ~1700 | 5–7 | ≤ 6.0 | 8–9 | 2007 |
| ACCORD [12] | ~10,000 | 4–8 (average 5.6) | < 6.0 | 7.0–7.9 (expected mean 7.5) | 2010 |
| ORIGIN[a] [19] | ~10,000 | 4–8 | FPG < 95 mg/dL (glargine) | < 7 A1c (standard care with no insulin) | 2008 |

[a] This study's glycemic target in the intervention group is FPG.

a 16% reduction in the relative risk of each of the primary endpoints for each of the randomized comparisons. More design details are published [8,9] and available on the website for the co-ordinating center, the George Institute for International Health in Sydney, Australia. In particular, 11,140 patients have been randomized and final results are expected in 2006, with an expected difference in HbA1c levels between randomized arms of 1%. Discussion on the website suggests that the difference between arms remains a challenge for the study [10].

*VADT*

The VADT (Veterans Affairs Diabetes Trial) started in December of 2000 with the goal of enrolling 1700 men and women 41 years of age or older with HbA1c level of 7.5% or higher despite therapy with oral agents or insulin. Volunteers are randomized to an intensive or standard treatment program and followed for 5 to 7 years for major CV events (MI, stroke, new or worsening congestive heart failure [CHF], amputation for ischemic diabetic gangrene, invasive intervention for coronary or peripheral arterial disease, and CV death). The study is designed to have 86% power to detect a 21% relative reduction in major CV events. In the intensive arm, the goal is to achieve an HbA1c level of 6% or less by sequential addition and titration of metformin, rosiglitazone, or evening intermediate NPH insulin or long-acting insulin glargine to achieve near-normal fasting glucose levels, and subsequent morning or multiple daily injections of short-acting insulins or other therapies as needed (eg, glimepiride and α-glucosidase inhibitors). In the standard arm, the goal is to avoid deterioration in HbA1c, keeping levels at 8% to 9%. The treatment algorithm for the standard group is less rigid and generally uses submaximal doses of oral agents. The investigators expect a difference between arms of 1.5% to 2% in HbA1c level. All patients receive an identical program of individualized diabetes mellitus education, medical nutrition therapy, blood pressure management, lipid management, aspirin therapy, and smoking cessation counseling per American Diabetes Association guidelines. Further details are available in a published methods paper [11].

*ACCORD*

The ACCORD trial (Action to Control Cardiovascular Risk in Diabetes) examines three independent medical treatment strategies for patients who have type 2 diabetes mellitus. At approximately 70 centers in the United States and Canada, 10,000 patients who have type 2 diabetes mellitus will be randomized in a double 2 × 2 design. All participants will be in the overarching trial that examines glycemic targets. Two subtrials will examine lipid and blood pressure hypotheses (see later discussion). The clinical question tested by the glycemia trial is: "in middle-aged or older people with type 2 diabetes who are at high risk for having a CVD event because of existing clinical or subclinical CVD or CVD risk factors, does a therapeutic strategy that targets a HbA1c level of < 6% reduce the rate of CVD events more than a strategy that targets a HbA1c level of 7% to 7.9% (with the expectation of achieving a median level of 7.5%)" [12]. Participants will be treated for 4 to 8 years (mean approximately 5.6 years) with main study results to be reported in 2010. The primary outcome measure of the trial is time to the first occurrence of a major CVD event (MI, stroke, or CV death), with the study designed to have 89% power to detect a 15% treatment effect of intensive glycemic control compared with standard glycemic control.

These three trials should answer definitively the clinical question of whether intensive glucose management will reduce the risk for CVD. Each seeks to achieve glycemic targets below levels reported in large clinical trials, and should inform the discussion about the appropriate targets for glycemic control and the magnitude of the risk of hypoglycemia involved. They also will examine effects on microvascular complications, quality of life, and cost-effectiveness. Because each uses different strategies to achieve different target levels of glycemic control in different populations, they will provide a rich set of data to drive future clinical recommendations. Although it is assumed widely that the hypotheses they seek to test are correct, there is substantial doubt as to the outcomes of these studies. Positive results will put tremendous pressure on health care systems to achieve even more stringent levels of control. Negative results will suggest the need to achieve HbA1c levels of approximately 7% to prevent microvascular complications, and that the attention vis-à-vis CV risk management should be on blood pressure, lipid, and thrombotic risk in diabetes mellitus.

**Trials examining glycemic management techniques**

The second fundamental question in diabetes management is whether particular glucose-lowering approaches, and more specifically insulin sensitizers, provide benefits beyond glucose lowering in managing CV risk. The possibility first was suggested based on the notion that insulin resistance is linked epidemiologically with components of the metabolic syndrome including dyslipidemia, dysglycemia, hypertension, a procoagulant state, vascular inflammation, endothelial dysfunction, and premature vascular disease [13,14]. Several small and medium-sized studies have supported the idea that insulin-sensitizing approaches could be superior to approaches that supplement deficient insulin secretion, suggesting improvements in markers of CV risk during treatment with metformin and thiazolidinediones when compared with other therapies. Furthermore, in the UKPDS, among overweight subjects, those randomly assigned to initial therapy with metformin (but not to insulin or sulfonylurea) demonstrated a reduction in diabetes mellitus–related deaths and MI compared with those treated with lifestyle intervention; the validity of this observation has been challenged because of the relatively limited sample size and the unusual responses in a subsequent subrandomization [7].

## BARI 2D

Arguably the BARI 2D study (Bypass Angioplasty Revascularization Investigation in Type 2 Diabetes) will offer the most straightforward assessment of this controversy. This multicenter study will recruit 2800 patients who have type 2 diabetes mellitus. Important inclusion criteria include age over 25 years and a coronary arteriogram showing one or more vessels amenable to revascularization with at least a 50% or greater stenosis and either objective documentation of ischemia or typical angina with at least a 70% coronary stenosis. Patients will be randomized in a 2 × 2 factorial design to examine two treatment strategies: one cardiac-related (coronary revascularization plus aggressive medical therapy versus aggressive medical therapy alone) and one diabetes-related (comparing insulin-providing versus insulin-sensitizing therapy). The diabetes treatment randomization will be to treatment focusing on providing more insulin, either endogenously, stimulated through the use of insulin secretagogues, or exogenously, administered through subcutaneous insulin injections, versus a strategy of increasing sensitivity to insulin by using metformin and/or one of the commercially available thiazolidinediones, pioglitazone or rosiglitazone. All patients will be treated with a target HbA1c level of < 7%. For those unable to achieve an HbA1c level less than 8% with one treatment strategy, crossover to combined treatment approaches will be used. The other randomization will examine two approaches to manage CVD: elective revascularization using surgery or catheter-based therapies combined with aggressive medical therapy versus aggressive medical therapy alone. The primary outcome for this trial is CV mortality. Additional outcomes include MI, angina, quality of life, employment, cost, and cost-effectiveness. Recruitment is expected to be complete in 2004, with results reporting in 2007 [15,16].

## PROactive

Several pharmaceutical industry–sponsored clinical trials will examine the effect of various specific agents on CV outcomes. Little published information on these trials is available. One exception is the PROactive study (Prospective Pioglitazone Clinical Trial in Macrovascular Events), which has reported its design and baseline characteristics. PROactive has randomized 5238 patients from 19 countries who have type 2 diabetes mellitus and a history of macrovascular disease to the addition of pioglitazone versus placebo onto existing baseline antidiabetic therapy. The primary endpoint is the time from randomization to occurrence of a new macrovascular event or death. The study was expected to reach its prespecified follow-up period depending on the rate of accrual of events in 2005 [17].

## RECORD

The RECORD study (Rosiglitazone Evaluated for Cardiac Outcomes and Regulation of Glycaemia in Diabetes) will randomize 6000 patients who have type 2 diabetes mellitus failing either sulfonylurea or metformin. Patients entering the study on metformin will be randomized to combination with sulfonylurea or rosiglitazone and patients entering the study on sulfonylurea will be randomized to combination with metformin or rosiglitazone. At 18 months, an interim analysis will examine glycemic control between arms. Patients will be followed for 6 years on rosiglitazone plus metformin or sulfonylurea versus metformin plus sulfonylurea or acarbose for combined CV endpoints [18].

## ORIGIN

The ORIGIN trial (Outcome Reduction with Initial Glargine Intervention) is a multicenter international study that will randomize in a $2 \times 2$ factorial design 10,000 people 50 years of age or older at high risk for CVD who have early type 2 diabetes mellitus as defined by an HbA1c level less than 9% if drug naïve or a lower A1c if treated with one oral antidiabetic agent. Persons who have prediabetes with either impaired fasting glucose (IFG) or with impaired glucose tolerance (IGT) will also be included. For the first randomization, patients will be assigned to treatment with insulin glargine titrated to normalize fasting glucose to < 95 mg/dL versus standard care, which generally will involve metformin or sulfonylurea therapy, at least in patients who have fasting hyperglycemia with sequential conventional tactics aiming at achieving A1c < 7%. Patients also will be randomized to a supplement of omega-3 polyunsaturated fatty acids versus placebo. The primary endpoint is combined CV morbidity and mortality outcomes, with projected study completion in late 2008 [19].

## NAVIGATOR

The NAVIGATOR trial (Nateglinide and Valsartan in Impaired Glucose Tolerance Outcomes Research) has randomized over 8000 individuals 55 years of age or older who have IGT in over 30 countries in a $2 \times 2$ factorial design to valsartan versus placebo and to the insulin secretagogue nateglinide versus placebo. Rate of progression from IGT to diabetes mellitus as an endpoint, will be examined 3 years after the last participant is randomized. After 1000 CV events have accrued, estimated to occur with 5 to 6 years of follow-up, composite CV morbidity and mortality outcomes will be examined as an endpoint [20,21].

## DREAM

The DREAM study (Diabetes Reduction Assessment with Ramipril and Rosiglitazone Medication) is similar in design to NAVIGATOR, but only examines CVD endpoints and surrogate CV risk markers as secondary endpoints. It also uses a $2 \times 2$ factorial design to examine the primary outcome if treatment with an angiotensin-converting enzyme (ACE) inhibitor (ramipril) or a thiazolidinedione (rosiglitazone) versus matched placebo can delay or prevent the development of type 2 diabetes mellitus in people who have IGT or impaired fasting glucose (IFG). Follow-up is planned until 2006 in the 5269 patients who have been recruited; further details are published [22].

Table 2 provides an overview of these six studies. In particular, the BARI 2D study should answer the question of whether sensitizer-based therapy is superior to insulin-supplementing therapy. The others likely will be confounded somewhat by differences in levels of glycemic control. To the extent that the studies involving patients who have prediabetes and early diabetes unlikely will exhibit much in the way of elevated glucose, even in the placebo or usual care groups, the effect of differences in glycemia on CVD risk should be minimized, isolating nonglycemic effects of these therapies to some extent. As a body of work, these studies will provide substantial new guidance for

Table 2
Studies of techniques of glycemic control and effects on cardiovascular disease

| Study [Ref.] | Population | No. of participants | Estimated completion | Randomized treatments | |
|---|---|---|---|---|---|
| | | | | 1 | 2 |
| BAR1 2D [15,16] | DM and coronary lesion | 2800 | 2007 | Insulin sensitizing | Insulin providing |
| PROACTIVE [17] | DM | 5238 | 2005 | Pioglitazone: | Placebo: |
| RECORD [18] | DM | 6000 | | metformin + rosiglitazone ± sulfonylurea | metformin + sulfonylurea ± acarbose |
| ORIGIN [19] | DM and prediabetes | 10,000 | 2008 | Glargine | Standard care |
| NAVIGATOR [20] | Prediabetes | 8000 | 2006 | Nateglinide | Placebo |
| DREAM [22] | Prediabetes | 5269 | 2006 | Rosiglitazone | Placebo |

Table 3
Other interventions under study

| Study [Ref.] | Randomized treatments | |
|---|---|---|
| | 1 | 2 |
| BARI 2D [15,16] | CABG or PCI + medical management | Medical management |
| FREEDOM [31] | CABG | Sirolimus-eluting stent |
| HPS II, SEARCH [35,36] | High-dose simvastatin | Lower-dose simvastatin |
| TNT [37] | High-dose atorvastatin | Lower-dose atorvastatin |
| IDEAL [35] | High-dose atorvastatin | Moderate-dose simvastatin |
| FIELD [38] | Fenofibrate | Placebo |
| ACCORD–Lipid [12] | Simvastatin + fenofibrate | Simvastatin + placebo |
| ACCORD–BP [12] | SBP < 120 mm Hg | SBP < 140 mm Hg |
| NAVIGATOR [20,21] | Valsartan | Placebo |
| DREAM [22] | Ramipril | Placebo |
| SPARCL (stroke) [39] | High-dose atorvastatin | Placebo |
| SHARP [40] | Simvastatin + ezetimibe | Simvastatin |
| ADVANCE [8,9] | ACE + thiazide | Placebo |
| Look AHEAD [42] | Lifestyle management for weight loss | Diabetes support and education |
| ORIGIN, ASCEND [19,46] | Omega fatty acid supplement | Placebo |
| SEARCH, HPS II [35,36] | Vitamins | Placebo |
| ASCEND [46] | Aspirin | Placebo |
| CARDia [32] | CABG | PCI |

optimal treatment strategies in approaching glycemic targets in type 2 diabetes mellitus.

**Studies examining nonglycemic therapies**

*Revascularization interventions*

Table 3 details other interventions under investigation. In the initial BARI trial, among the diabetic subgroup a dramatic advantage of coronary artery bypass graft surgery (CABG) was observed compared with percutaneous coronary intervention (PCI) with angioplasty; the benefit was seen primarily in the more than 80% of patients who had an internal mammary artery graft [23]. Since then, several advances have been made in the management of the acute coronary syndrome [24,25], the medical management of coronary disease [26], and the techniques of PCI (eg, stents and, most promisingly, drug-eluting stents) [27–30].

This leaves questions regarding the appropriate management of the patient who has diabetes mellitus and flow-limiting coronary disease. Two trials will explore these issues robustly. The BARI 2D trial will explore whether intensive medical management or intensive medical management plus bypass surgery or PCI improves survival in patients who have type 2 diabetes mellitus [15,16].

The FREEDOM trial (Future Revascularization Evaluation in Patients with Diabetes Mellitus: Optimal Management of Multivessel Disease) will compare CABG to PCI using the drug-eluting stents in diabetic patients who have multivessel disease, following the patients for 5 years to examine mortality as the primary endpoint. Investigators at 100 sites will recruit 2300 patients who have diabetes mellitus and at least two stenotic lesions in at least two major epicardial coronary arteries amenable to either PCI or surgical revascularization over 18 months. Intermediate endpoints, quality of life, neurocognitive function, and cost-effectiveness also will be examined. FREEDOM is planned to be complete in 2010 [31]. The CARDia trial (Coronary Artery Revascularization in Diabetes) is a smaller study of 600 individuals in the United Kingdom and Ireland that began recruitment in 2002 and is similar in intent to FREEDOM. CARDia addresses the hypothesis that optimal PCI is not inferior to modern CABG in patients who have diabetes with multivessel or complex single-vessel coronary disease assuming that the PCI 1-year event rate is 9%. The primary endpoint of death, nonfatal MI and nonfatal stroke will be assessed at 1 year and the population followed for a total of 5 years for a broad range of secondary endpoints [32].

*Lipid interventions*

No area of CVD research in diabetes has received more attention than lipid management. Numerous studies in primary prevention and secondary intervention with statins and fibrate lipid-lowering agents are underway [33]. The guidelines regarding lipid management are in flux based on the rapidly evolving landscape of clinical trials that have recently and soon will be reported. Recent guidelines discussed elsewhere in this issue reinforce prior recommendations that in high-risk patients like those who have type 2 diabetes mellitus, the low-density lipoprotein cholesterol (LDL-C) goal is less than 100 mg/dL, but suggest that in the highest risk patients, such as those who have acute coronary syndrome or diabetes mellitus and clinical CVD, further lowering to an LDL-C level of 70 mg/dL or less is "a therapeutic option, ie, a reasonable clinical strategy" [34].

A remaining question is how low should one go in managing lower risk patients who have diabetes mellitus? Several trials addressing this will report in the near future: HPS II (Heart Protection Study II), IDEAL (Incremental Decrease in Endpoints through Aggressive Cholesterol Lowering) [35], SEARCH (Study of the Effectiveness of Additional Reductions in Cholesterol and Homocysteine) [36], and TNT (Treating to New Targets) [37]. Each examines the effect of different levels of low-density lipoprotein (LDL) control with high and moderate doses of one agent (HPS II, SEARCH, and TNT) or different levels of control obtained in comparisons of two agents (IDEAL). Approximately 40,000 patients are randomized in those studies, which will report starting in 2005.

Despite fairly robust demonstration of the role of gemfibrozil in the management of CV risk, issues have arisen regarding the safety of combining statins and fibrates. Thus, with many statin trials documenting the usefulness of statins to reduce CVD in virtually every clinical situation, questions exist regarding the appropriate role of fibrates in the management of CVD risk in diabetes mellitus. The FIELD trial (Fenofibrate Intervention and Event Lowering in Diabetes) randomized 9795 people who had type 2 diabetes with average total cholesterol (115–250 mg/dL) and elevated triglyceride to high-density lipoprotein cholesterol (HDL-C) ratio (> 9.2) or triglyceride level greater than 88 mg/dL to fenofibrate or placebo. FIELD is expected to

report on the primary endpoint, CVD death and nonfatal MI, in 2005 [38]. FIELD should establish the role of fenofibrate, a newer fibrate with fewer issues regarding drug interactions with statins.

The ACCORD study has a lipid substudy in which approximately 5800 participants also will be randomized to fenofibrate or placebo in the context of therapy with simvastatin to achieve LDL levels of approximately 100 mg/dL or lower. The ACCORD lipid study will answer whether a treatment strategy that uses a fibrate to raise HDL-C and lower triglycerides and a statin to treat LDL reduces the rate of CVD events compared with a strategy that uses only a statin for treatment of LDL-C, establishing the safety and efficacy of statin-fibrate combination therapy [12].

Finally, several studies will examine the role of lipid management in particular clinical situations common in patients who have diabetes mellitus, such as the SPARCL study (Stroke Prevention by Aggressive Reduction in Cholesterol Levels), which will evaluate the effects of atorvastatin in the setting of transient ischemic attack [39], and the SHARP study (Study of Heart and Renal Protection), which will examine the effect of simvastatin versus simvastatin/ezetimibe combination therapy in dialysis patients [40].

*Blood pressure interventions*

Many have argued that blood pressure management is the most important aspect of diabetes care because it has tremendous impact on the risk for microvascular and macrovascular complications [41]. Strictly speaking, the current systolic blood pressure goal of less than 130 mm Hg has not been tested formally in clinical trials because that level has not been achieved and sustained in studies; the diastolic goal of less than 80 mm Hg is better studied.

ACCORD's second substudy will randomize 4200 participants to two levels of blood pressure control to answer whether, in the context of good glycemic control, a therapeutic strategy that targets a systolic blood pressure (SBP) of < 120 mm Hg reduces the rate of CVD events compared with a strategy that targets a SBP of < 140 mm Hg. The ADVANCE trial also has a blood pressure substudy in which patients will be randomized to a fixed low-dose combination of the ACE inhibitor perindopril and the thiazide diuretic indapamide or matching placebo to produce a difference in blood pressure between arms.

NAVIGATOR and DREAM will examine the roles of valsartan, an angiotensin-receptor blocker, and ramipril, an ACE inhibitor, on CVD.

*Lifestyle interventions*

Another crucial question in diabetes management is whether lifestyle intervention can affect CVD outcomes. Lifestyle management is a critical component of all diabetes management. Short-term studies of medical nutrition therapy, physical activity, and comprehensive lifestyle approaches have improved the control of classic CVD risk factors as well as intermediate markers of CVD risk, such as C-reactive protein. However, no long-term large-scale study of intentional weight loss has been powered to examine CVD endpoints.

Look AHEAD (Action for Health in Diabetes) will examine CVD events for up to 11.5 years in patients 45 to 74 years of age who have type 2 diabetes mellitus and a body mass index $\geq 25$ kg/m$^2$ [40]. Patients will be randomized to a 4-year intensive weight-loss program (calorie restriction and physical activity) or to "diabetes support and education." With planned recruitment of 5000 patients at 16 centers over 2.5 years, the study is designed to provide a 0.90 probability of detecting an 18% difference in major CVD event rates between arms.

*Miscellaneous interventions*

Finally, a related topic is whether antioxidant vitamins, B-vitamin supplementation to lower homocysteine, or various fatty acids can promote CV health in diabetes mellitus. All have been associated with lower risk in epidemiologic analysis, although no consistent findings have emerged from large-scale randomized trials in people who have diabetes mellitus [42–44]. The ORIGIN trial will evaluate the effect of omega fatty acids in patients who have diabetes mellitus and prediabetes and CVD risk factors; ASCEND (A Study of Cardiovascular Events in Diabetes) also will do so in patients who have diabetes mellitus in the setting of primary prevention in a 2 × 2 factorial design in which the second randomization will be to aspirin, 100 mg/d, versus placebo [45]. SEARCH and HPS II will randomize subjects to various vitamin supplements or placebo to examine whether these relatively inexpensive interventions provide clinical benefit to reduce CVD as well.

**Summary**

There has been an explosion of interest in CVD and diabetes mellitus because of the epidemic nature of the diseases and their tight epidemiologic link. Clinical trials over the past decade have built substantial evidence for the role of lipid management, blood pressure control, and antiplatelet therapy in managing risk for CVD in patients who have diabetes mellitus. The many clinical trials underway will not only hone existing recommendations by establishing appropriate targets and techniques for lipid and blood pressure management, but also should demonstrate the role and most appropriate techniques for management of glycemia, flow-limiting coronary lesions, and obesity.

**Acknowledgments**

The authors wish to thank the Council for the Advancement of Diabetes Research and Education (CADRE) for assistance in gathering information for this study.

**References**

[1] Buse J, Raftery L. What we think and what we know. Diabetes Care 2002;25:1876–8.

[2] ClinicalTrials.gov. Available at: http://clinical trials.gov/ct. Accessed on August 8, 2004.

[3] American Diabetes Association. Standards of medical care in diabetes. Diabetes Care 2004;27(Suppl 1): S15–35.

[4] American Association of Clinical Endocrinologists and the American College of Endocrinology. The American Association of Clinical Endocrinologists medical guidelines for the management of diabetes mellitus: the AACE system of intensive diabetes self-management—2002 update. Endocr Pract 2002;8(Suppl 1):40–82.

[5] Third Joint Task Force of European and Other Societies on Cardiovascular Disease Prevention in Clinical Practice. European guidelines in cardiovascular disease prevention in clinical practice. Eur J Cardiovasc Prev Rehabil 2003;10(Suppl 1):S1–78.

[6] UK Prospective Diabetes Study Group. Intensive blood-glucose control with sulphonylureas or insulin compared with conventional treatment and risk of complications in patients with type 2 diabetes (UKPDS 33). Lancet 1998;352(9131):837–53.

[7] UK Prospective Diabetes Study Group. Effect of intensive blood-glucose control with metformin on complications in overweight patients with type 2 diabetes (UKPDS 34). Lancet 1998;352(9131):854–65.

[8] ADVANCE Management Committee. Study rationale and design of ADVANCE: action in diabetes and vascular disease—preterax and diamicron MR

controlled evaluation. Diabetologia 2001;44(9): 1118–20.

[9] Rationale and design of the ADVANCE study: a randomised trial of blood pressure lowering and intensive glucose control in high-risk individuals with type 2 diabetes mellitus. Action in diabetes and vascular disease: preterax and diamicron modified-release controlled evaluation. J Hypertens Suppl 2001;19(Suppl 4):S21–8.

[10] The George Institute for International Health. Available at: http://www.iih.org. Accessed March 12, 2004.

[11] Abraira C, Duckworth W, McCarren M, et al for the participants of the VA Cooperative Study of Glycemic Control and Complications in Diabetes Mellitus Type 2. Design of the cooperative study on glycemic control and complications in diabetes mellitus type 2. Veterans Affairs Diabetes Trial. J Diabetes Complications 2003;17(6):314–22.

[12] ACCORD purpose. Available at: http://www.accordtrial.org/public/purpose.cfm. Accessed August 8, 2004.

[13] Kunhiramen BP, Jawa A, Fonseca VA. Potential cardiovascular benefits of insulin sensitizers. Endocrinol Metab Clin N Am, in press.

[14] Reaven GM. Compensatory hyperinsulinemia and the development of an atherogenic lipoprotein profile: the price paid to maintain glucose homeostasis in insulin-resistant individuals. Endocrinol Metab Clin N Am, in press.

[15] Sobel BE, Frye R, Detre KM. Burgeoning dilemmas in the management of diabetes and cardiovascular disease. Rationale for the Bypass Angioplasty Revascularization Investigation 2 Diabetes (BARI 2D) Trial. Circulation 2003;107(4):636–42.

[16] Bypass Angioplasty Revascularization Investigation in Type 2 Diabetics (BARI 2D). Available at: http://www.clinicaltrials.gov/ct/show/NCT00006305?&order = 1. Accessed August 8, 2004.

[17] Charbonnel B, Dormandy J, Erdmann E, et al on behalf of the PROactive Study Group. The prospective pioglitazone clinical trial in macrovascular events (PROactive): can pioglitazone reduce cardiovascular events in diabetes? Study design and baseline characteristics of 5238 patients. Diabetes Care 2004;27(7):1647–53.

[18] Homan R. Shifting the paradigm from stepwise to early combination therapy. Available at: http://www.cmeondiabetes.com/pub/shifting.the.paradigm..from.stepwise.to.early.combination.therapy..php. Accessed August 8, 2004.

[19] The ORIGIN Trial (Outcome Reduction with Initial Glargine Intervention). Available at: http://www.clinicaltrials.gov/ct/show/NCT00069784?&order = 1. Accessed August 8, 2004.

[20] Pratley R. NAVIGATOR: nateglinide and valsartan in impaired glucose tolerance outcomes research. Available at: http://www.novartis.se/products/diabetes/Pratleypermissions.ppt. Accessed August 8, 2004.

[21] Novartis Pharmaceuticals USA. Novartis announces largest diabetes and cardiovascular disease prevention trial with starlix and diovan. Available at: http://www.pharma.us.novartis.com/newsroom/press Releases/releaseDetail.jsp?PRID = 141&checked = y. Accessed August 8, 2004.

[22] Gerstein HC, Yusuf S, Holman R, et al. Rationale, design and recruitment characteristics of a large, simple international trial of diabetes prevention: the DREAM trial. Diabetologia 2004;47(9): 1519–27.

[23] The BARI investigators. Influence of diabetes on 5-year mortality and morbidity in a randomized trial comparing CABG and PTCA in patients with multivessel disease: the Bypass Angioplasty Revascularization Investigation (BARI). Circulation 1997;96: 1761–9.

[24] Fox KA. Management of acute coronary syndromes: an update. Heart 2004;90(6):698–706.

[25] Schwartz GG, Olsson AG, Ezekowitz MD, et al. Myocardial Ischemia Reduction with Aggressive Cholesterol Lowering (MIRACL) Study Investigators. Effects of atorvastatin on early recurrent ischemic events in acute coronary syndromes: the MIRACL study: a randomized controlled trial. JAMA 2001;285(13):1711–8.

[26] Pitt B, Waters D, Brown WV, et al. Aggressive lipid-lowering therapy compared with angioplasty in stable coronary artery disease. Atorvastatin versus Revascularization Treatment Investigators. N Engl J Med 1999;341(2):70–6.

[27] Levine GN, Kern MJ, Berger PB, et al. American Heart Association Diagnostic and Interventional Catheterization Committee and Council on Clinical Cardiology. Management of patients undergoing percutaneous coronary revascularization. Ann Intern Med 2003;139(2):123–36.

[28] Beyar R. Novel approaches to reduce restenosis. Ann N Y Acad Sci 2004;1015:367–78.

[29] Kokolis S, Cavusoglu E, Clark LT, et al. Anticoagulation strategies for patients undergoing percutaneous coronary intervention: unfractionated heparin, low-molecular-weight heparins, and direct thrombin inhibitors. Prog Cardiovasc Dis 2004;46(6): 506–523.

[30] Bavry AA, Kumbhani DJ, Quiroz R, et al. Invasive therapy along with glycoprotein IIb/IIIa inhibitors and intracoronary stents improves survival in non-ST-segment elevation acute coronary syndromes: a meta-analysis and review of the literature. Am J Cardiol 2004;93(7):830–5.

[31] FREEDOM Trial: Future Revascularization Evaluation in Patients with Diabetes Mellitus: Optimal Management of Multivessel Disease. Available at: http://www.clinicaltrials.gov/ct/show/NCT00086450. Accessed August 15, 2004.

[32] Kapur A, Malik IS, Bagger JP, et al. The Coronary Artery Revascularization in Diabetes (CARDia) trial: background, aims, and design. Am Heart J 2005;149:13–9.

[33] Deedwania PC, Hunninghake DB, Bays H. Effects of lipid-altering treatment in diabetes mellitus and the metabolic syndrome. Am J Cardiol 2004; 93(11A):18C–26C.

[34] Grundy SM, Cleeman JI, Merz CN, et al. Coordinating Committee of the National Cholesterol Education Program; National Heart, Lung, and Blood Institute; American College of Cardiology Foundation; American Heart Association. Implications of recent clinical trials for the National Cholesterol Education Program Adult Treatment Panel III guidelines. Arterioscler Thromb Vasc Biol 2004; 24(8):e149–61.

[35] Deanfield JE. Clinical trials: evidence and unanswered questions—hyperlipidaemia. Cerebrovasc Dis 2003;16(Suppl 3):25–32.

[36] MacMahon M, Kirkpatrick C, Cummings CE, et al. A pilot study with simvastatin and folic acid/vitamin B12 in preparation for the Study of the Effectiveness of Additional Reductions in Cholesterol and Homocysteine (SEARCH). Nutr Metab Cardiovasc Dis 2000;10(4):195–203.

[37] Waters DD, Guyton JR, Herrington DM, et al. TNT Steering Committee Members and Investigators. Treating to New Targets (TNT) Study: does lowering low-density lipoprotein cholesterol levels below currently recommended guidelines yield incremental clinical benefit? Am J Cardiol 2004;93(2):154–8.

[38] FIELD. Available at: http://www.ctc.usyd.edu.au/trials/cardiovascular/field.htm. Accessed August 15, 2004.

[39] Amarenco P, Bogousslavsky J, Callahan AS, et al. SPARCL Investigators. Design and baseline characteristics of the stroke prevention by aggressive reduction in cholesterol levels (SPARCL) study. Cerebrovasc Dis 2003;16(4):389–95.

[40] Study of Heart and Renal Protection (SHARP): study summary. Available at: http://www.ctsu.ox.ac.uk/~jobs/SHARPsummary.doc. Accessed August 12, 2004.

[41] Snow V, Weiss KB, Mottur-Pilson C. Clinical Efficacy Assessment Subcommittee of the American College of Physicians. The evidence base for tight blood pressure control in the management of type 2 diabetes mellitus. Ann Intern Med 2003;138(7): 587–92.

[42] Ryan DH, Espeland MA, Foster GD, et al. Look AHEAD (Action for Health in Diabetes): design and methods for a clinical trial of weight loss for the prevention of cardiovascular disease in type 2 diabetes. Control Clin Trials 2003;24(5): 610–28.

[43] Stanger O, Herrmann W, Pietrzik K, et al. Clinical use and rational management of homocysteine, folic acid, and B vitamins in cardiovascular and thrombotic diseases. Z Kardiol 2004;93(6): 439–53.

[44] Jha P, Flather M, Lonn E, et al. The antioxidant vitamins and cardiovascular disease. A critical review of epidemiologic and clinical trial data. Ann Intern Med 1995;123(11):860–72.

[45] Montori VM, Farmer A, Wollan PC, et al. Fish oil supplementation in type 2 diabetes: a quantitative systematic review. Diabetes Care 2000;23(9): 1407–15.

[46] ASCEND: a randomised study of aspirin and of omega-3 fatty acid supplementation for the primary prevention of cardiovascular events in diabetes. Available at: http://www.ctsu.ox.ac.uk/ascend/. Accessed September 6, 2004.

# Index

*Note:* Page numbers of article titles are in **boldface** type.

0733-8651/05/$ - see front matter © 2005 Elsevier Inc. All rights reserved.
doi:10.1016/S0733-8651(05)00014-7

*cardiology.theclinics.com*

# Changing Your Address?

Make sure your subscription changes too! When you notify us of your new address, you can help make our job easier by including an exact copy of your Clinics label number with your old address (see illustration below.) This number identifies you to our computer system and will speed the processing of your address change. Please be sure this label number accompanies your old address and your corrected address—you can send an old Clinics label with your number on it or just copy it exactly and send it to the address listed below.

We appreciate your help in our attempt to give you continuous coverage. Thank you.

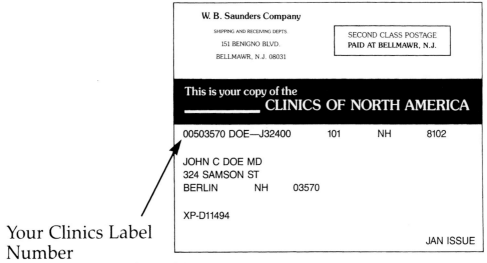

**W. B. Saunders Company**

SHIPPING AND RECEIVING DEPTS.
151 BENIGNO BLVD.
BELLMAWR, N.J. 08031

SECOND CLASS POSTAGE
PAID AT BELLMAWR, N.J.

This is your copy of the
CLINICS OF NORTH AMERICA

00503570 DOE—J32400        101        NH        8102

JOHN C DOE MD
324 SAMSON ST
BERLIN        NH        03570

XP-D11494

JAN ISSUE

## Your Clinics Label Number

Copy it exactly or send your label
along with your address to:
**W.B. Saunders Company, Customer Service**
Orlando, FL 32887-4800
Call Toll Free 1-800-654-2452

Please allow four to six weeks for delivery of new subscriptions and for processing address changes.